Also by Harris H. McIlwain, M.D., and
Debra Fulghum Bruce, Ph.D.

The Pain-Free Back
Pain-Free Arthritis
The Fibromyalgia Handbook
Stop Osteoarthritis Now
Winning with Heart Attack
Winning with Back Pain
Winning with Chronic Pain
Winning with Osteoporosis
The 50+ Wellness Program
The Super Calcium Counter
The Unofficial Guide to Conquering Impotence
Bone Boosters
The Osteoporosis Cure
Super Aspirins

Also by Debra Fulghum Bruce, Ph.D.

The 24-Hour Turnaround
Miracle Touch
Overkill
The Sinus Cure
Making a Baby
Eat Right to Stay Young
The Snoring Cure
The Unofficial Guide to Alternative Medicine
Breathe Right Now

Reversing Osteopenia

Reversing Osteopenia

- THE DEFINITIVE GUIDE
- TO RECOGNIZING
- AND TREATING
- EARLY BONE LOSS
- IN WOMEN OF ALL AGES

Harris H. McIlwain, M.D.,
and Debra Fulghum Bruce, Ph.D.,

with Laura McIlwain Cruse, M.D.,
and Kimberly Lynn McIlwain, M.D.

AN OWL BOOK

HENRY HOLT AND COMPANY · NEW YORK

Owl Books
Henry Holt and Company, LLC
Publishers since 1866
175 Fifth Avenue
New York, New York 10010
www.henryholt.com

An Owl Book® and ® are registered trademarks of
Henry Holt and Company, LLC.

Library of Congress Cataloging-in-Publication Data

McIlwain, Harris H.
   Reversing osteopenia : the definitive guide to recognizing and
treating early bone loss in women of all ages / Harris H. McIlwain
and Debra Fulghum Bruce with Laura McIlwain Cruse
and Kimberly Lynn McIlwain.—1st ed.
     p. cm.
   Includes bibliographical references and index.
   ISBN-13: 978-0-8050-7622-6
   ISBN-10: 0-8050-7622-0
   1. Osteopenia—Popular works. 2. Women—Health and hygiene—
Popular works. I. Bruce, Debra Fulghum, date. II. Title.

RC931.O716M38 2004
616.7'16—dc22   2004047528

Henry Holt books are available for special promotions and
premiums. For details contact: Director, Special Markets.

First Edition 2004

Designed by Victoria Hartman

Printed in the United States of America
10 9 8 7 6

To our mothers and grandmothers
Cordelia Bryant McIlwain
and Jewel Holden Fulghum

Contents

Introduction

Picture someone who needs to be concerned about bone loss. Do you immediately think of a frail woman with stooped posture? Perhaps you envision an elderly woman shuffling along the sidewalk with cane in hand. The truth is, bone loss affects millions, and not just little frail older women. Each of the following women was recently diagnosed with bone loss at our clinic:

- Marilee, age thirty-two, a healthy athlete who competes in marathons around the world
- Shawn, age thirty-nine, a mother of two who underwent a surgical hysterectomy four years ago and opted not to take estrogen replacement
- Caroline, age twenty-six, a vegan since early college days who also takes prednisone (a corticosteroid medication) for rheumatoid arthritis
- Reagan, age forty, a petite attorney with a lengthy history of eating disorders including bulimia and exercise obsession

Would you ever associate these young women with bone loss and fractures? Do you see yourself in the descriptions above?

We've treated these young women—and thousands more—for a type of bone loss called osteopenia. This forerunner to osteoporosis is a silent but deadly condition that can lead to painful and deforming fractures. Osteopenia begins to rob bones during the most productive time of a woman's life—from childbearing years to perimenopause. The good news is we've found that treating osteopenia before a broken bone happens is as effective as treating high blood pressure before a stroke or high cholesterol before a heart attack.

We wrote this book to give all women the latest information about America's escalating bone loss crisis and what they can do today to guarantee healthy, strong bones. We also wrote this book to increase an awareness of osteopenia among younger women. In fact, a critical study reported at the American Alliance for Health, Physical Education, Recreation and Dance meeting in August 2002 showed that almost 20 percent of college-age women already have osteopenia, which sets them up for early painful fractures. Today 34 million Americans, or 55 percent of women fifty years of age and older, have osteopenia, which puts them at increased risk of developing full-blown osteoporosis and painful fractures.

Our Goals for This Book

In writing this book, we had two major goals:

1. To show millions of women of all ages how osteopenia can easily be diagnosed and reversed before its only symptoms—broken bones—appear.

2. To provide realistic, age-specific ways women and children can optimize their bone strength early on to avoid or reverse osteopenia and subsequent fractures altogether.

It's important to understand that there is no "one-size-fits-all" approach to keeping bones strong. That's why we are passionate about writing one of the first books on osteopenia, so all women can have an effective and balanced approach—*one tailored to your unique situation*—to keeping bones strong for a lifetime.

The problem with osteopenia is that there are no warning signs until you fracture a bone. If left undiagnosed and untreated, osteopenia can lead directly to osteoporosis, in which the bones become thin, weaker, and fracture easily. Once osteoporosis is diagnosed, there are treatments to increase the amount of bone and lower the chances of fractures. But the new bone is often not as strong as the original bone. This means the risk for fractures is lower than if you got no treatment at all, but it's higher than if the bone was normal.

There's no reason to wait until your bones have irreversibly weakened to take action! Detecting osteopenia with a bone density test (see page 19) is easy. From there, making a plan to to prevent disfiguring and painful fractures is simple and straightforward.

If you're wondering why osteopenia is a topic of real concern for young women today, consider this: many years ago, it was not thought important to treat hypertension (high blood pressure) because there were no obvious consequences. Over the past forty to fifty years, it has been shown that treating high blood pressure lowers the risk of stroke years later. Thirty years ago, blood cholesterol was not considered abnormally high until it exceeded 300. Now we know that treating cholesterol levels at 200 can prevent heart attacks years later.

It has been shown that the connection between bone loss and fractures is stronger than the connection between high blood pressure and stroke, or between high blood cholesterol and heart attack. You can stop and reverse osteopenia before a fracture—*if you take action early in life.*

We know that osteopenia can be *halted and reversed* long before women enter menopause and face early fractures because of the dramatic decline of estrogen levels. Awareness is crucial. Once women are aware of their personal risk for osteopenia and the direct consequences of painful or debilitating fractures, they can make plans with their doctors to start the 5-Step *Bone-Building Program* detailed in this book.

Our Introduction

Who are we? Harris McIlwain (hereafter Dr. Harris) is a practicing rheumatologist and founding partner of Tampa Medical Group, P.A., located on Florida's sunny Gulf Coast. An internationally renowned arthritis specialist, Dr. Harris has treated thousands of patients with pain-related ailments over the past thirty years. Because he also diagnoses and treats all stages of bone loss daily, he is dedicated to finding new treatment breakthroughs to help patients prevent further bone loss and the subsequent debilitating fractures.

In addition to being a rheumatologist, Dr. Harris is a dedicated father. He and his wife, Linda, have raised six children in Tampa. As a staunch believer in the health benefits of exercise for all ages, Dr. Harris has coached youth soccer teams for more than twenty years.

For this revealing how-to guide, Dr. Harris is joined by his two oldest children: Dr. Laura McIlwain Cruse (Dr. Laura) and Dr. Kimberly McIlwain (Dr. Kim), both board certified in internal medicine and completing fellowships in rheumatology. As avid runners, both Dr. Laura, who is married to Hugh Cruse and is the mother of two-year-old Bennett, and Dr. Kim have an intense commitment to educating young women about ways to keep bones strong and healthy.

Together, we're going to educate you about osteopenia, a little-known problem that is becoming commonplace even among young women today. We'll discuss the latest research on preventing and treating bone loss, and success stories from our rheumatology practice, in the hope that you will use this information to improve the health of your bones.

Why We Are Passionate about Stopping Bone Loss

We are conventionally trained physicians and have witnessed the tremendous benefits of bone-saving medications and high-tech procedures. Yet we also know that easy lifestyle modifications, such as giving up cigarettes and limiting alcohol, combined with complementary and alternative medicine (CAM) therapies such as dietary changes, vitamins and minerals, and regular exercise, can halt and even reverse bone loss. This realization has helped us personalize our 5-Step *Bone-Building Program*, making it highly accessible for *every* woman, no matter what her age or health history.

Dr. Harris's story: It's obvious that prevention and early treatment of any problem is better than waiting for the consequences. Treating high blood pressure is easier and cheaper than treating strokes and treating high blood cholesterol is easier and more effective than treating heart attacks with stents and coronary bypass.

Bone loss results in fractures—spines, hips, wrists, shoulders, and ankles—and costs over $17 billion each year. This enormous amount does not include the cost of losing one's independence. In fact, one-third of hip fracture patients are unable to resume their established daily routines. Many require nursing home care. There is even a higher risk of death after a hip fracture.

Throughout my years in medical practice, I've believed in finding a health problem while it's easy to prevent and treat—and this goes for osteopenia, too. I emphasize with all my patients that we need to find low bone mass when there are no outward signs or feelings—while it's easily treated. Then, follow the 5 steps in the *Bone-Building Program* and prevent unfortunate consequences.

In this book, Laura, Kim, and I will provide you with the latest information on how to protect yourself—and your family—from osteopenia and painful fractures. We'll explain how you can assess your personal risk for this painful and disfiguring disease and then outline an age-specific program to help you be your own bodyguard and keep your bones strong no matter what your health history.

It sounds simple—and it is. Taking proven steps to keep bones strong is so much easier than dealing with debilitating fractures, medications, therapy, lifestyle changes, and even loss of independence or death.

Dr. Laura's story: Since I was a small girl, exercise has always been an important part of my life. From years of team sports to mainly running today, I strongly believe that exercise helps my mind, body, and spirit—and my bones, too!

Now, as I try to balance marriage, parenting, and career, time is very important to me. However, I've realized that a well-balanced diet and a consistent exercise program are the cornerstones of staying strong and healthy. My health is essential to my family's well-being too. For me—as well as for my family. After all, if I get sick, who will fill in for me when our baby cries at two A.M.? Or, if I'm completely exhausted, who will make key decisions about patients' health when I'm on call at night? I see *no* volunteers!

As a doctor, I see young women who smoke and diet very strictly. Many do not realize the risks these habits pose to their bones. I always encourage the women to strengthen their bones as much as they can right now—to protect against problems later on in life. There are many medical conditions, as well as the medications used to treat these ailments, that can result in thin bones. That's why it's important to participate in your health care to limit the side effects and remove the possible confounding factors altogether.

In short, I believe that all women should be role models—for their children, spouses, and those around them. If we set good, strong examples, we can train the next generation to live healthily too. I know it's a big responsibility, but the reward of living an active life—the rest of your life—is certainly well worth it.

Dr. Kim's story: So many problems in life silently build up, only to declare themselves many years later when things are beyond our control. I find that this is true particularly for young women, who often put their health on a back burner in order to pursue higher education, a career, or a family. In fact, the time many younger women should be using to exercise and invest in their bone health is usually spent taking care of other people and working on an endless to-do list.

Through talking with patients and peers, I know that some women even feel guilty blocking time for themselves—for daily exercise or learning about proper nutrition that can prevent illness. Instead, many rely on "quick fixes"—habits that help them cope in the short term, such as relying on fast food and take-out meals or postponing exercise in order to work another hour or spend more time writing e-mail to friends. Smoking is another behavior some women use to cope with the stress of their hectic lives. Some women use cigarettes and very-low-fat diets (thus, typically low calcium) to help control weight without having to exercise—both of which can lead to weak bones and osteopenia.

It disturbs me that sometimes the answer to a strong and healthy life is often only clear in hindsight. That's why I am committed to teaching all young women the key to reversing osteopenia before it's too late. The key, as we discuss in this book, is to spend the time *early on in life* building strong bones. By following the recommended diet and exercise plan in the 5-step *Bone-Building Program*, the prevention of osteopenia is only part of the ongoing reward. You'll also experience increased energy, a sense of control, and greater mental strength.

I hope you learn from the insight and recommendations in this book, and then share the book with other women. Perhaps increased awareness about osteopenia starts with just one woman, but my dream is that word will spread and as a group we'll all grow stronger together. Our overall goal is to grow as a group of strong, highly motivated, and successful women.

We'll Give You Personalized Guidance

Whether you're in your 20s, 30s, 40s, or beyond, we will give you age-specific guidance with our 5-step *Bone-Building Program* to help you assess your bone strength and reverse osteopenia. We want to place you, the reader, at center stage by focusing on your personal risk factors for osteopenia. As you read through the book, you will see that it quickly moves beyond a description of the problem of osteopenia to page after page of personalized self-help tips that you can use right now to boost your bone strength, stay healthy, and, most important, dramatically reduce your chance of fractures.

Here's how we'll accomplish this:

In Step 1, *Baby Your Bones*, we'll give you the facts you need to know about osteopenia—what it is, how it is diagnosed, why it's a serious concern, and more. We will detail the specific risk factors for osteopenia and explain how a simple, painless bone density test can let you and your doctor know the condition of your bones. We'll share some eye-opening statistics to show you the global magnitude of the problem of bone loss and then give you age-specific ways in which you can be your own bodyguard against osteopenia.

Step 2, *The Bone-Building Workout*, is perhaps the most important step in this book. Here we'll help you focus on your personal exercise plan to keep bones strong. There are many options for bone-building exercises, and we want you to find the exercises that you enjoy doing that are also proven to strengthen bone mass and prevent disease.

You'll evaluate your daily diet and make changes to improve the condition of your bones and overall health in Step 3, *Feed Your Bones*. A host of vitamins, minerals, and other key nutrients are vital for bone health. We'll explain the eating plan and give you age-specific guidelines for calcium, vitamin D, phosphorus, and other nutrients. If you're allergic to dairy or adhere to a vegetarian or vegan diet, we'll give you lists of nondairy foods that are high in calcium and other bone-boosting nutrients.

Step 4, *Take Strong Steps to Prevent Fractures*, is a must-read for every woman—no matter what her age. In this key step, we'll discuss the problem of "bone-robbers," such as smoking and excessive drinking of alcohol. We'll also teach you some proven ways to make easy changes at home to prevent falls—the number one cause of hip fracture.

In Step 5, *An Integrative Medicine Approach*, we clarify the hormone replacement therapy (HRT) debate for anyone considering it, and give you some safe bone-building medicines that can be used to increase bone density. We'll also acquaint you with some commonly used naturopathic remedies to keep bones strong. From natural dietary supplements like over-the-counter calcium tablets to soy isoflavone pills, there's a long list of readily available and effective approaches to increasing bone strength.

In chapter 6, we introduce some *Special Situations* that can increase your understanding of bone loss and its prevention and treatment for different segments of the population. In this section, we discuss:

- Children and teens
- Postmenopausal women
- Men and bone loss

- Spine fractures and back pain
- Surgery and fractures

We believe that eating the right nutrients is crucial in achieving optimal bone strength. Our fifty bone-building recipes in chapter 7 use the foods recommended in Step 3. Not only are the recipes easy to make, but they are also delicious and your family will enjoy them.

Finally, every woman will benefit from the stretches and range-of-motion and strengthening exercises explained in chapter 8. These exercises are easy to learn, can be done in the privacy of your home, and allow you to increase repetitions as you are physically able.

Here's to Strong Bones . . . All of Your Life!

So, how strong are your bones? Could years of low-calorie or deprivation dieting have depleted your bones of the necessary nutrients to stay strong? Could a sedentary lifestyle devoid of exercise have resulted in a decrease in bone density? What about the medications you've taken over the years? Could these have robbed your bone density?

There's only one way to find out the state of your bones—and that's to assess your bone strength in Step 1, and then take the necessary measures to keep them strong (Steps 2 to 5). To that end, our *Bone-Building Program* will provide you with all the information and tools you need to find a balanced approach that best suits you and your family.

Now let's get started!

Dr. Harris, Dr. Laura, and Dr. Kim

Reversing Osteopenia

CHAPTER 1

Step 1: Baby Your Bones

Today more than ever, you must be the guardian of your own health. That means making informed decisions regarding early detection, prevention, and treatment of illness to keep yourself and your family healthy. While treating disease is critical, especially in the early stages when treatment works best, there is a compelling case supported by a host of scientific data that the prevention of any health problems should be your primary goal.

Before we talk about specific ways you can baby your bones and prevent or reverse osteopenia or low bone mass, we need to explain the epidemic problem of bone loss and how the resulting painful and disfiguring fractures can rob you of your youthful appearance and an active, productive life.

Diagnosis: Osteopenia

Patient's Name: Christie
Age: 41
Risk factors: History of low-calorie dieting, avoidance of dairy, thyroid disease

Forty-one-year-old Christie had never heard of osteopenia until she had a bicycle accident and injured her wrist. This active mother of three was riding bikes with her family when her front tire hit a curb, and she was thrown onto the hard pavement. She broke her fall with her hands but luckily did not receive a fracture. However, because she had a history of thyroid disease, dairy allergies, and years of low-calorie dieting—all key risk factors for osteopenia—we did a bone density test at our clinic. The results of her test revealed that she had early bone loss or osteopenia with the bone density of a woman ten years older.

Patient's Name: Wendy
Age: 30
Risk factors: Family history (grandmother), excessive exercise, amenorrhea, low body weight

---

Wendy, age thirty, came to our clinic after her gynecologist raised concern about her low body weight and ordered a bone density test. As an avid marathon runner, Wendy was thin, muscular, and appeared to be the picture of health. But this young woman also dieted excessively and experienced amenorrhea (loss of menstrual periods)—key risk factors for osteopenia and fractures. Wendy told us that the first time she heard of bone loss was when the family discussed her grandmother's sudden death after complications from a hip fracture. "I thought thin bones were something older women got, not active people my age," she said after hearing the diagnosis of osteopenia.

Patient's Name: Janie
Age: 39
Risk factors: Early menopause (surgical), lack of estrogen replacement, sedentary lifestyle

---

Janie had never been an exerciser and had an early menopause with hysterectomy in her early thirties because of fibroid tumors. She discovered her bone loss problem when she and some friends took advantage of a free screening—a heel bone density test—at a mall health fair. Three of the five women were found to have low bone mass. Because Janie did not supplement with estrogen hormone therapy after her surgery, she did not receive the protective effect on bones of estrogen hormone treatment. She later had a DEXA test which confirmed she had osteopenia.

Understanding the Female Athlete Triad

The *female athlete triad* is a constellation of medical conditions that are becoming increasingly common in women athletes. Specifically, these are eating disorders, amenorrhea (lack of menstrual periods), and osteopenia or low bone mass. Athletes who compete in gymnastics, dancing, swimming, skating, and running are at high risk for the female athlete triad, as they strive to appear lean and fit.

We know that more female athletes have amenorrhea than women in the general population. Amenorrhea is associated with decreased estrogen levels, which may be the cause of osteopenia or low bone mass. Low-calorie diets are usually the first predictor of eating disorders. Excessive exercise or exercise obsession can be another sign of an eating disorder. Each of these three problems must be medically evaluated and treated to ensure a good outcome.

Defining Bone Loss

Are you surprised to hear that young women today are faced with bone thinning and fractures? Don't be! Osteopenia has been labeled the "young women's silent epidemic" by some experts because there are no warning signs. Such trendy behavior for young women as social drinking, smoking, drinking excessive amounts of coffee and diet colas, deprivation dieting, and lack of bone-strengthening exercise are all having a devastating effect on young bones. Even taking some forms of birth control may increase the risk of bone loss. For example, Depo-Provera (medroxyprogesterone acetate), an injectable contraceptive that prevents ovulation (the release of the egg by the ovary), causes the body to stop producing estrogen and progesterone. Both hormones are important for bone strength since estrogen slows down bone loss, and progesterone boosts bone growth.

Osteopenia is every woman's concern—no matter what her age or health status—as this is the first stage preceding full-blown osteoporosis or severe bone loss. Moreover, fractures don't wait until you have osteoporosis. The risk of fractures increases with decreases in bone density. Once you have just *one fracture*, you are at a greater risk for more fractures. The good news is that osteopenia can be prevented or reversed before debilitating fractures occur.

What Is Osteopenia?

Osteopenia is thinning of bones that can be detected by a simple bone density test (see page 19) long before there is the severe bone loss and fracture risk of osteoporosis. In osteopenia, the bone density is lower than normal but not yet full osteoporosis.

Many patients are confused when they hear that they have osteopenia. After all, the media has focused on full-blown osteoporosis for years with its resulting stooped posture and painful fractures. However, a diagnosis of osteopenia also means a greater risk of fractures. Studies indicate that patients with osteopenia sustain more fractures than patients with osteoporosis. It makes sense that the best time to take steps to reverse bone loss, strengthen bones, and prevent fractures is when osteopenia is found.

A Major Risk for Fractures

So, if osteopenia is a growing problem in the United States, why haven't you read much about it? Mainly, because *doctors are just now beginning to learn how to deal with bone loss*—just like they're learning to deal with heart disease in women. For instance, a decade ago, heart disease was not diagnosed in women until after a near fatal heart attack and loss of heart muscle. Doctors simply did not associate heart disease with women, even though it is now regarded as the single greatest health risk for women.

Today, we know that keeping a regular check on body weight, blood pressure, and cholesterol can help prevent a woman's heart attack altogether, and both doctors and patients recognize the need to take preventive measures with lifestyle changes.

Similarly, doctors are realizing that osteopenia is a major risk for the development of fractures. It is a warning sign that alerts you to take action before permanent damage is done from bone thinning. New estimates suggest *that half of all women over the age of forty-five are now affected by low bone mass, including 90 percent of women over age seventy five*. Moreover, those numbers continue to grow. That's why it's important to understand osteopenia and your personal risk factors in order to prevent or reverse bone loss before fractures occur.

At menopause, there is a dramatic decline of estrogen, which causes rapid bone loss, leading to devastating hip fractures. Having the strongest bones possible *before you enter menopause* is the best weapon against debilitating fractures. While the emphasis in the medical community has been on postmenopausal women as prime targets of bone loss awareness campaigns, many—including the authors!—believe the target should include younger women, especially those who have time to reverse osteopenia before it results in debilitating fractures.

Once bone has been lost in full-blown osteoporosis, treatment may not build bone that is as mechanically strong as the original bone. In other words, even if the bone density test results improve, the bone may never be as strong as it was before.. This makes the finding of osteopenia a *life-saving warning sign*.

While it is more common for women to suffer from fractures after menopause because of the dramatic drop in estrogen levels and the effect on bone, the process of bone loss begins much earlier. The stage is set for osteopenia early in life—*in your teens, 20s, 30s, and 40s.* The problem is there are *no* noticeable symptoms of bone loss until you experience a sudden, painful fracture or substantial loss of height because of a vertebral fracture. By then, bones have become so weak that even mild stress like bending over, lifting a bag of groceries, or coughing can cause a fracture, horrific pain, and immobility.

We believe that the fracture you want to prevent is *the first one*. By identifying women with risk factors for osteopenia early in life—while they can still make lifestyle changes to strengthen bones—we might prevent millions of fractures altogether.

Imagine if all the women who suffer from painful hip fractures now could have had this lifesaving information twenty years ago! The key to living a strong life is simple: early detection and taking a few easy prevention steps to baby your bones years before bone loss and fractures occur.

Understanding Fractures

With osteopenia, bones become thin and weak, which makes them easier to break. Though painful, the break will usually heal. Yet, as long as the bones are thin and weak, they are increasingly susceptible to fractures and the subsequent immobility or even death. In fact, in adults, a grave predictor of bone problems is a previous fracture that occurred after a minor fall. If you had a fracture because of weak bones, your risk of another fracture is 2 to 20 times greater than someone who has never had a fracture.

Half of all Americans will break a bone before age sixty-five. Now, if such fractures only affected fingers or toes, it would be inconvenient but not terribly limiting. However, bone loss commonly attacks with painful vengeance, severely limiting the activities of daily life.

According to the National Osteoporosis Foundation (NOF), bone thinning is responsible for more than 1.5 million fractures each year. More than 300,000 hip fractures happen annually. While hip fracture is the most devastating fracture associated with bone loss, vertebral (spine) fracture is the most common, with over 750,000 each year.

Fractures can be painful; they also cause deformities and are expensive. For example, fractures, especially when they affect the spine, can cause deformities such as the dowager's hump. The cost of hip fractures alone—both direct (hospitalization, surgery, and doctors' visits) and indirect (lost time from work)—exceeds $17 billion annually. This cost will only sky-rocket . . . unless we take action early on to prevent and reverse osteopenia. The number of fractures will also escalate over the next few years as the projected population over age sixty-five increases. One study recently predicted 4.5 million annual hip fractures worldwide in the year 2050.

None of this has to happen to you. Doctors can treat and even reverse osteopenia and help you build stronger bones and end fractures forever.

Hip Fractures

"Aren't I a bit too young for a bone density test? Fractures only happen in the elderly," Suzi, a thirty-six-year-old woman with a history of eating disorders and exercise obsession, shared her concerns as we scheduled her for a bone density test. Untrue! While general bone loss among women commonly begins in the perimenopausal period (the years prior to menopause), bone loss from the hip can begin even earlier. Suzi's bone density score showed osteopenia and was lower than that of other women her age. Because of this, Suzi was at higher risk for future fractures.

If you know someone who has had a hip fracture, then you have reason to be concerned about your own bone health. Hip fractures are very serious injuries, often a turning point, beyond which independent living is no longer possible. Perhaps you have a family member who was active and living alone—until she fell and broke her hip. For those who suffer hip fracture, recovery can be difficult as they face hospitalization, surgery, and months of painful, exhausting, and expensive therapy.

The National Osteoporosis Foundation (NOF) estimates that *a woman's risk of hip fracture is equal to her combined risk of breast, uterine, and ovarian cancers*. Nearly one-fourth of hip fracture patients age fifty and older die in the year following their fracture, and one-fourth of those who were ambulatory before their hip fracture require long-term care afterward.

Although there are several different areas in the hip that may break, most breaks are called hip fractures. These usually require surgery, since without surgery it takes six weeks or more of bed rest for fractures to heal. With surgery, the patient can usually be up and walking within a few days.

The operation to correct these fractures is expensive, usually $35,000 to $40,000 or more. Along with this cost comes the higher risk of other serious medical problems such as blood clots, heart attack, pneumonia, and stroke. The worst cost is that many of these victims immediately lose their independence.

Studies confirm that 95 percent of hip fractures result from falls. Weight-bearing and strengthening exercises (chapter 2) and the ancient art of tai chi (see page 38) are excellent ways to keep your body toned and flexible and your bones strong, so you can stay balanced and avoid falls and fractures no matter what your age.

Spinal Fractures

Spinal fractures affect more than 50 percent of all women. Significant changes in the spine from bone thinning are common. By age seventy-five, *more than 50 percent* of women have had a fracture in their spine with an estimated half-million vertebral fractures occurring annually. The most common deformity from bone loss, called the dowager's hump, happens in the upper part of the spine (see figure 1.1).

Only about one-third of vertebral fractures produce symptoms. Generally, fractures in the lower spine are associated with more pain and loss of function than fractures in the upper spine, and multiple fractures are more problematic than a single fracture.

Each fractured vertebra becomes shorter, usually by about one-quarter inch, and the spine bends forward. This gradually makes the person appear stooped over and results in decreased height. The loss of height may not even be noticed until you are measured in your doctor's office. In fact, the most common cause of loss of height as we age is bone loss. The stooped-over posture can make the abdomen more prominent. One of our patients said that she went from a height of 5'4" as a young woman to 4'11" at age seventy-five with full osteoporosis (see figure 1.2).

As bones become thinner and weaker, the effort required to hold the body erect while standing or walking may be enough to cause a fracture. Bending can greatly stress the spine, often putting pressure equivalent to several times the weight of the body on the back. This pressure leads to fractures in weakened bones.

After age forty-five, the most common cause of height loss is shortening

Figure 1.1

The Spine

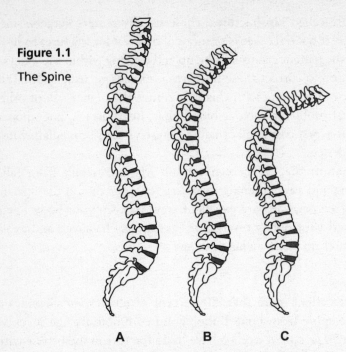

A   B   C

A. Normal spine   B. Spine with early fractures
C. Spine with osteoporosis and more fractures

of the bones of the spine by bone thinning. However, doctors should suspect bone loss in any person—no matter what her age—who loses height. When osteopenia affects the spine, fractures can happen in one of the vertebral bones. If each fracture in the spine causes about one-quarter-inch loss of height, after many fractures there may be a loss of several inches in total height. Treatments, as described in Step 5, have been shown to greatly lower the risk of more fractures and help *delay* the shortening and deformity of the spine that cause the stooped posture.

When bone loss is present and weakens the bones, it is a wonder that sufferers do not experience more fractures in the spine. Science tells us that lifting an 86-pound object from the floor can place 700 pounds or more of force on the back. One fifty-one-year-old woman said that she had her first spinal fracture, along with weeks of excruciating pain, after merely opening her bedroom window. During the first week she was completely bedridden from the pain.

Fractures in the spine cause back pain that can be severe, making it difficult to stand, walk, sit, or lift. In some cases, the pain can be so excruciating as to make the smallest movement difficult and almost any position

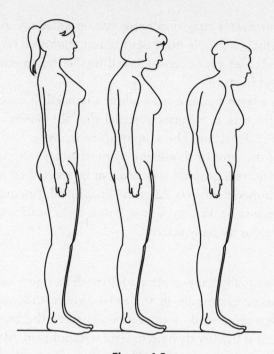

Figure 1.2

The dowager's hump

uncomfortable. It can also cause loss of independence, as we can no longer care for our families and ourselves.

Once a spinal fracture occurs, the pain may worsen when you try to walk, bend, or lift. This pain commonly makes it hard to sleep well at night. You may feel penetrating pain when you cough or sneeze. (Pain from a spinal fracture does not usually travel down the legs; so if you have this feeling, let your doctor know.)

Sometimes you may fracture more than one bone in the spine, resulting in pain that lasts longer than a few weeks. If pain is severe for longer than a few days, check with your doctor. There may be an additional problem in the spine. If you notice a change in your bladder or bowel habits, such as loss of control, then call your doctor to be sure no other serious problems are present.

Wrist and Shoulder Fractures

The wrist and the shoulder are common places for early bone loss with more than *200,000 wrist fractures annually*. Fractures in these bones usually happen after a fall, such as with Christie's bicycle accident, discussed on page 1. Your doctor may find bone loss on an X ray. As we recommended to Christie, a simple bone density test, discussed on page 19, can be administered to let your doctor know if further treatment is needed to prevent the next fracture.

If you have a wrist fracture as an adult, you need to have a bone density test. The fracture is a common signal that the bones are becoming thinner; the next signal could be a hip or spine fracture.

Fractures of the wrist or shoulder may need an operation to repair, but most do not require a hospital stay and can be treated on an outpatient basis by an orthopedic surgeon. After the bones heal, you may need to see a physical therapist or do exercises at home to be sure you do not lose usage of these areas for daily activity.

Pelvic Fractures

Pelvic fractures usually happen after a fall, with an injury to the bones of the pelvis, causing great pain in the pelvis, lower abdomen, and groin areas. This often requires days or weeks in bed or the hospital. After a pelvic fracture, it is frequently hard to walk without pain. After a few days to a week, most patients can stand. Then, after a few more days, they can walk again. If you have a fracture of a bone in the pelvis, you need to have a bone density test. If bone loss is found, steps must be taken to prevent more fractures, especially a hip fracture.

The Emotional Side of Fractures

Not only are multiple fractures disfiguring and painful, they are a significant emotional burden. After one fracture you may become anxious and

---

Fracture Fast Facts

- One in two women and one in four men over age fifty will have an osteoporosis-related fracture in their lifetime.
- Osteoporosis is responsible for more than 1.5 million fractures annually, including:

  – More than 300,000 hip fractures
  – More than 750,000 vertebral fractures
  – More than 250,000 wrist fractures
  – More than 300,000 fractures at other sites

fearful about the possibility of others. Many people limit activity or exercise and become socially isolated. Depression and feelings of hopelessness are commonplace, especially if activities become limited.

Some women with chronic pain are well aware that they are depressed. The signs are obvious: uncontrollable tearfulness, a persistent sad or anxious mood, feelings of hopelessness, guilt, or irritability, loss of interest in nearly all activities, decreased energy, difficulty concentrating or making decisions and, in severe cases, thoughts of death or suicide. Loss of self-esteem can also occur due to the disabling and disfiguring aspects of the fractures.

What Your Doctor May Not Have Told You

In a national survey of 1,000 women age thirty and older, published in the *Washington Times,* 7 out of 10 women said their doctors had never said anything about bone loss prevention, treatment, or detection. Less than one-fourth of women with a strong family history of thin bones said their doctor recommended early detection with a bone density test. Almost all of our patients say they'd never heard of osteopenia until we brought it up!

Other frightening findings show that *more than half of the women who break a bone after age fifty*—which is the number one symptom of bone loss—say their doctor has never recommended that they be tested with a bone density test. These women were untested—and untreated. We believe that a bone density test after a fracture is as important as an electrocardiogram for a woman who has suffered a heart attack or a blood glucose test for a suspected diabetic.

It's thought that the average primary care physician sees about one hundred patients each week who have various stages of bone loss. Yet doctors are so busy treating other problems that they miss unseen bone loss. In addition, until recently, there was little doctors could do to detect bone loss. Today there is something they can do. Our job as health care professionals is not just to "fix the fracture," leaving millions of women with osteopenia untreated, but to treat and reverse this early stage of bone loss.

The challenge for all of us is to detect low bone mass as early as possible, when it is most treatable. Now, with new diagnostic tools, every woman who suspects low bone mass or who has *one of the risk factors* for osteopenia, discussed on page 15, can quickly and inexpensively have a bone density test (see page 19).

We want you to be aware of the negative emotions that often coincide with the early stages of bone loss, fracture, and chronic pain, so you can take control. The *Bone-Building Program* will help to ease depression, as you become more physically active and find solutions to reverse or prevent bone loss and your risk of fractures. There are also excellent antidepressants available that both improve pain and have a positive mood effect. In fact, many chronic pain patients have received excellent relief from a combination of antidepressants and other pain-relieving drugs.

Understanding the Bone Cycle

Before we can talk about a proven program to reverse osteopenia and painful fractures, we need to explain the underlying physiology of how bone is built and lost during our lifetime.

Childhood: Bone Building Exceeds Bone Loss

Bone is not a lifeless structure. Rather, it is complex, living tissue. As if on schedule, our bodies naturally break down old bone and rebuild new bone, an intricate process called remodeling. In children, more bone is built than removed, so during this life stage, bones become larger and stronger. In fact, the skeleton may reach about 95 percent of its peak amount of bone by age twenty. Some experts believe that during childhood up to the early twenties, young women can increase their bone mass by as much as 20 percent—a critical factor in protecting against bone loss and fractures. We believe that the more bone you store, the more you will have to draw on later in life.

Age 30 to 35: Bone Loss Equals Bone Building

Around age thirty to thirty-five, the amount of bone our bodies break down begins to catch up with the amount of bone our bodies are building. Sometime during this period, the bone mass removed equals the bone mass built.

Perimenopause: Bone Loss Exceeds Bone Building

Perimenopause is the period before menopause when estrogen levels first start their decline. At this time (about age thirty-five to forty-five), the mass of bone removed may begin to exceed the mass of bone built. It is at this time that osteopenia disrupts the natural bone-building cycle, resulting in a decrease in net bone mass.

Menopause: Bone Loss Accelerates

Menopause is a normal life transition, starting with perimenopause. Perimenopause and menopause are not medical diseases. These are natural times during which your body undergoes a number of changes in metabolism, hormone production, and the length and frequency of menstrual periods, among other things.

At menopause, the hormonal changes disrupt this bone-building cycle again. Specifically, the natural decline in estrogen at menopause speeds up the breakdown of bone. During the five to ten years after menopause, there is a greatly accelerated loss of bone mass in women. Within the first five years after menopause, some women have lost up to a startling *25 percent of their bone density*.

This may be difficult to comprehend for active women in midlife who take their good health for granted. Yet reports say more than 30 percent of perimenopausal women (late 30s to late 40s) have osteopenia and a startling 20 percent of women in their 40s have osteoporosis. Sadly, it is estimated that *only 10 to 15 percent of those who have bone loss actually know they have it*. Many women don't arrive at this knowledge until they fracture a bone, and even then many are still not aware of the problem.

How Healthy Are Your Bones?

"So, when will I have a fracture? What signs should I look for?" Lynn's concern was apparent when she was given the results of her bone density test. Then she added, "Isn't osteopenia a problem my mother or grandmother should worry about—not a thirty-eight-year-old woman with two preschoolers?"

When women ask "if" or "when" they will have a bone fracture, we always tell them that we cannot predict the hour, minute, or second a fracture might happen. Nonetheless, we *can* identify things they do or health conditions they have that put them at greater risk. Whether you develop osteopenia at all depends on various risk factors such as the thickness of your bones early in life, as well as your family history, age, overall health, diet, physical activity, and lifestyle later in life.

To see how healthy your bones are, put the following on your bone-building "to-do" list:

To-Do #1: Assess your personal risk for osteopenia.
To-Do #2: Schedule a bone checkup.
To-Do #3: Ask your doctor about a bone density test.

To-Do #1: Assess Your Personal Risk

Risk factors are those habits or histories that alone and together increase the likelihood you'll develop a medical condition. For instance, if you are overweight, smoke cigarettes, and have high blood pressure, your risk for heart disease is greater than a nonsmoker's who is at an optimal weight with normal blood pressure. In the case of osteopenia, some risk factors are inherited, such as a family history of bone loss and fractures. Some are tied to your individual medical history. Women with thyroid disease, those who experience an early menopause with hysterectomy, or who have irregular menstrual periods may develop osteopenia at an early age. Other risk factors are the result of lifestyle choices, such as lack of weight-bearing exercise, avoiding dairy products, or smoking.

No matter what they are, the specific risk factors for osteopenia do their damage in silence. You have no idea that you are losing bone density until you have a fracture, after which your risk for more fractures is greatly increased. We've treated many young women with osteopenia who outwardly appear be the picture of health. Many are muscular athletes, yet still have weak bones.

The good news is that early recognition of risk factors and following the 5-step *Bone-Building Program* can keep you from suffering with debilitating fractures in years to come.

In our practice, we've treated women ages nineteen to over a hundred. The younger our patients are, the harder it is for them to believe they are at risk for osteopenia and fractures. Maybe you're the same way. You're not old enough to have osteopenia! Or maybe you believe—mistakenly, as our patients have learned—that bone loss is a natural part of the aging process to be expected and accepted. While bone loss does happen with age, it should *never be accepted* and can be prevented before painful and deforming fractures occur.

As you review the following risk factors, keep in mind that risk factors for osteopenia add up. For instance, having three risk factors is definitely worse than having one or two. Still, no matter what your age, the more risk factors you address now, the more you reduce your risk for osteopenia and future fractures.

12 Signs Your Bones Need Attention

The best way to approach your personal risk of osteopenia is to get a piece of paper and write down any of the following 12 signs (risk factors) that mean your bones might need attention. After you've made your personal risk factor list, check off those that you can control with bone-boosting changes, starting today. Talk to your doctor about the other signs or risk factors to see if further steps need to be taken to help prevent osteopenia and fractures.

1. ***Low body weight.*** Your weight influences your bone density. Some women maintain a low body weight through low-calorie dieting in order to look thin and so put themselves at increased risk for bone loss. For example, a woman who weighs less than 127 pounds is 10 times more likely to have lower bone density than a woman who weighs 150 pounds or more. The risk of bone loss increases when the percent of body fat becomes low. Women who diet excessively to maintain a low body weight often eliminate dairy products from their diet, losing their primary source of calcium—a vital source of bone strength.

2. ***Genetics.*** Did your mother or grandmother have stooped posture or height loss? This increases your risk of bone loss. Your risk of osteopenia and fractures is strong if your mother or grandmother had bone loss or fractures. The genetic predisposition may account for up to 60 to 80 percent of bone mass, while environmental factors account for the remaining 20 to 40 percent. That's why it's important to ask about your mother's and grandmother's bone health history. Families often share lifestyle habits such as diet, lack of exercise, or smoking cigarettes. You can change all of this and by doing so rewrite your bone health future.

3. ***Race.*** While non-Hispanic white and Asian women over fifty years old have a higher risk of bone loss and non-Hispanic black women over fifty have a lower incidence of bone loss, some recent findings are cause for concern for all women . When large numbers of women were tested, it was found that low bone mass is much more common than once believed in all ethnic groups, including African Americans. It is estimated that about 50 percent of white women over age fifty have osteopenia. And studies now confirm that 55 percent of Hispanic women, 65 percent of Asian women, 58 percent of Native American women, and 38 percent of African-American women have low bone mass and are at greater risk for fractures.

4. ***Age.*** The risk for bone loss increases with age. An estimated 90 percent of women over the age of seventy-five have experienced a bone fracture.

Low bone mass appears in about 50 percent of women in their 50s, 66 percent of women in their 60s, 86 percent of women in their 70s, and 93 percent of women over eighty.

5. *Early menopause.* The longer your body is exposed to estrogen, the lower your risk of bone loss and fractures. For instance, if you started menstruating late in your teenage years or if you experience menopause before your late 40s, your body produces less estrogen, putting you at higher risk for osteopenia.

6. *Previous fractures.* If you have had a fracture as an adult, your risk of more fractures is much higher. If you have a fracture in the spine (vertebral fracture), the risk is about 1 in 5 that you will have another one *within a year* if you don't take action. And a spine fracture can *double* your risk of a hip fracture! This is enough reason to have a bone density test and take lifestyle measures to reverse osteopenia.

7. *Certain medications.* The use of corticosteroid medications, such as prednisone or other cortisone derivatives, often leads to premature bone loss (these medications are common treatments for chronic conditions such as asthma, rheumatoid arthritis, and psoriasis). In fact, if you take these medications for more than three months, your risk for bone loss is high enough that experts recommend taking medication to prevent bone loss as well.

In addition, diuretics, antacids, chemotherapy, hormone therapy for cancer, lithium, and some medications for seizures can also sap the bones of calcium.

8. *Lifestyle habits.* Certain lifestyle habits such as smoking can lead to bone loss. On average, smoking doubles the risk of bone loss. The fastest-growing group of smokers in the United States are girls between the ages of twelve and eighteen. Younger women—under forty—often smoke in response to stress or to stay slim. Smokers also tend to have a higher consumption of alcohol, may be less physically active, often skimp on nutrition—all of which can lead to early bone loss. Smoking cigarettes seems to have an anti-estrogen effect on the bones, and women who smoke tend to go through menopause at least two years earlier than nonsmokers.

Excess consumption of alcohol can also lead to bone loss, since it reduces bone formation and interferes with the body's ability to absorb calcium. Drinking more than three alcoholic drinks per day can cause rapid bone loss. Moderate consumption by itself does not raise the risk.

9. *Avoidance of dairy products.* Calcium is the key mineral that makes up the dense structure of bone. The effect of calcium on bone health is most crucial during youth, when bones are growing quickly. In fact, it is thought that calcium deficiencies in childhood can account for a

5 to 10 percent difference in peak bone mass and can significantly increase the risk for hip fracture in later life. Some studies say that less than 25 percent of adolescent females are actually getting the calcium they need each day through foods or supplements. This deficit comes at a critical time in a woman's life—just before bone mass peaks. During menopause, especially in the first few years, calcium has a less dramatic effect since the rate of bone loss accelerates during this time. Still, getting ample calcium through foods and natural dietary supplements is vital to ensure the body has enough bone-building ability.

Calcium must be replenished daily through dietary measures or supplementation or the body will be deficient. Although the optimal level of calcium intake has not been clearly established, it is recommended that daily calcium intake be at least 1,200 milligrams (mg) in premenopausal women and 1,500 mg in postmenopausal women. (See Step 3, page 60, for specific information on how to boost calcium in the diet. In Step 5, page 98, we give specific information on increasing calcium in the diet with natural dietary supplements.)

Vitamin D is usually categorized as a fat-soluble vitamin, although it actually functions as a hormone in the body. Vitamin D helps to activate calcium and phosphorus (another key mineral for keeping bones strong) into the bloodstream. This is especially important as menopause approaches. When the body is depleted of vitamin D or has an insufficient supply, the blood levels of calcium and phosphorus plummet as well. Your body turns to the bones for replenishing this mineral and bone loss increases.

10. *Irregular menstrual periods.* Amenorrhea (the absence of menstrual periods) and other menstrual irregularities are also associated with an increase in fracture risk (see Understanding the Female Athlete Triad, page 3). Amenorrhea can occur because of strenuous exercise, and is common in female athletes, especially gymnasts and others who train hard but keep their body weight low. Women with amenorrhea experience significant reductions in estradiol, the primary form of estrogen. In most cases, amenorrheic premenopausal women have lower bone mineral density, particularly in the spine, than women who have normal menstrual cycles. The young female athlete who appears to be in top physical condition often has the highest risk of osteopenia and fracture, particularly if she experiences an eating disorder and loss of menstrual periods.

11. *Thyroid problems.* Too much thyroid hormone can cause bone loss. This condition occurs when the thyroid is overactive (hyperthyroidism)

or when excessive thyroid hormone medication is used to treat an under-active thyroid (hypothyroidism). A blood test called thyroid-stimulating hormone (TSH) can monitor hormone levels accurately and help women get the right amount of thyroid medication.

12. *Rheumatoid arthritis.* This type of inflammatory arthritis is most common in young women. It causes joint pain, swelling, and stiffness and can do permanent damage to the joints. Rheumatoid arthritis, as well as the cortisone medications often used for treatment, both raise the risk of bone thinning and fractures.

Risk Factors for Osteopenia

1. Low body weight
2. Lifestyle habits (smoking, excessive drinking)
3. Avoidance of dairy products
4. Irregular menstrual periods
5. Genetics (family history)
6. Previous fractures
7. Race (Caucasian or Asian)
8. Early menopause (surgical or natural)
9. Age
10. Certain medications
11. Thyroid problems
12. Rheumatoid arthritis

To-Do #2: Schedule a Bone Checkup
When patients schedule a visit to our clinic, we ask them to bring to the appointment a written list of any personal health concerns. We realize that it's easy to forget the problems you've had in the past or the names of medications you've taken, especially when you're busy juggling kids, a career, and other commitments. Yet, to make an accurate bone assessment, we need to know as much about your personal health history as possible. Before your visit, write down the following:

1. Any health problems or concerns
2. Symptoms you've noticed (loss of height, back pain, posture problems)
3. Past illnesses and treatment (see page 17)
4. Your family history of bone loss and fractures

5. Medications you are taking now; medications you've taken in the past
6. Your lifestyle habits (diet, exercise, smoking, alcohol consumption)
7. Your diet history (low-calorie diet, intake of dairy)
8. Questions you have about osteopenia and fractures

During the examination, your doctor will talk to you about any past or present symptoms or health problems. If your doctor doesn't ask the "right" questions, then openly volunteer any helpful information, as this may prevent you from having a fracture in the future. If necessary, your doctor might recommend a bone density test.

To-Do #3: Ask Your Doctor about a Bone Density Test
Amanda was a thin young woman who was extremely health conscious. At age thirty-one, she was a nonsmoker and vegetarian, and even grew her own vegetables in a small garden behind her condominium complex. She carefully watched her weight during pregnancy, gaining only twenty pounds, and then lost this weight within six weeks after delivery.

Amanda said she'd never given a thought to bone loss and figured that it was something only elderly women faced. Then she had a bone density scan, which clearly indicated osteopenia. Not only was Amanda thin, but her bones were thin and more fragile, putting her at double the risk of fracture. We explained to Amanda that unless she took immediate bone-strengthening steps, she could be at risk of developing fractures long before she reached an advanced age—the stress on her bones of simply picking up her preschooler could result in a fracture.

If you want to avoid having one of the more than 1.5 million fractures that occur each year from bone loss, a bone density test can help you plan ahead. The bone density test evaluates the strength of the bones in your body by measuring a small part of one or a few bones. The areas most commonly measured include:

- The hip
- The lumbar spine (in the lower back)
- The heel

The DEXA Test
The most widely used and accurate test at this writing is the DEXA (Dual Energy X-ray Absorptiometry) test of the hip and lower spine. This

simple and accurate test can be the first step in deciding whether medications are needed to treat bone loss.

The DEXA measures bone mineral density and converts the measurement into a standardized value called a *T score* (see table 1.1). Higher T-score values mean stronger bones. These results show how your bone density compares to a twenty-five-year-old woman. The test is painless, takes about ten minutes, and exposes you to only a fraction of the radiation needed for a chest X ray.

Warning Signs for Osteoporosis

- Any fracture after age 40
- Bone density test T score below −2.5
- Loss of height
- Dowager's hump (curve in the upper back)
- Back pain

The heel sonogram test. If you can't get a DEXA test, another option is the heel sonogram test (see table 1.2). This test is quick, taking only three to four minutes. It's painless and often done at shopping malls and free health screenings. The heel sonogram can be done while you are sitting in a chair and is useful for letting you know if you definitely need to have the more accurate DEXA test.

Table 1.1 Taking Action with a DEXA Test

T Score	Diagnosis	Action to Take
Greater than −1.0	Normal	Prevention steps needed
Between −1.0 and −2.0	Osteopenia	Talk with your doctor*
Below −1.5	Osteopenia	Talk with your doctor*
Below −2.0	Osteoporosis	Talk with your doctor*

*Depending on your age and other risk factors (page 15), treatment such as medications might be necessary.

There are other ways to measure bone mass and diagnose osteopenia, but they are less often used or more expensive. If you need one of these other tests your doctor can help you decide and make the specific plans for testing.

We remind patients that the T-score measurement may be different with different machines used and with different brands of machines. So, especially when you compare your T score to a previous result, keep in mind that what seems like a big difference may not actually be a real change. This is complicated, but just be sure that you talk with your doctor when you compare several T-score results over time—this may save much needless worry, especially when it appears that your bone mass has decreased. We often see patients who worry and add or change medications because of an apparent worsening of bone density test results. Many times this is simply the result of different ways of testing and *not* a sign of declining bone health.

Table 1.2 Heel Sonogram Test

T Score	Diagnosis	Action to Take
0 to −1.0	Possible osteopenia	Talk to your doctor. You *may* need to confirm the results with a DEXA test to check for osteopenia.
Below −1.0	Possible osteoporosis	Talk to your doctor. You *should* confirm the results with a DEXA test.

Normal results: If your bone density test score is normal, this means that you are not yet at a higher risk of fracture. Take the opportunity to talk with your doctor about prevention measures, including eliminating risk factors over which you have control (see page 15). Make sure you follow Steps 2 to 5 in the *Bone-Building Program*, including doing the right type of exercise (Step 2), eating a healthy diet filled with bone-strengthening foods (Step 3), maintaining lifestyle habits that keep bones strong (Step 4), and taking medications, if needed, and bone-strengthening supplements such as calcium and vitamin D (Step 5).

Osteopenia: If the bone density test shows osteopenia, then steps must be taken to help prevent fractures. This goes for men as well as women, since up to 30 percent of bone loss patients are men. Your doctor might recommend calcium and vitamin D supplementation, dietary changes, increasing exercise, and, depending on your age, using specific bone-building medications (see page 111). Treatment can effectively increase bone density, and it is well established that if you increase your bone density, you also lower your risk of painful and disfiguring fractures. If you have relatives with bone loss and fractures yet have no other risk factors, the bone density test can put your mind at ease.

Who needs a DEXA test? You might be wondering if everyone should have a bone density test, just to play it safe. *The answer is no.* But in certain situations, a bone density test is absolutely critical.

The universal public health directives are vague and unclear at best.

The current recommendation by the U.S. Preventive Services Task Force (USPSTF) of the National Osteoporosis Foundation (NOF) is that women have bone density tests at sixty-five and older—when many already suffer from some form of significant bone loss. Current research estimates that only about 12 percent of women over the age of sixty-five actually have gotten a bone scan.

One fact is clear—if you *don't* get a bone density test, you probably won't be treated even if your bones are thinning. Then eventually you may develop a fracture, get an X ray, and discover osteoporosis. But in fact many patients who have a fracture still aren't diagnosed or treated. Many patients, even after a hip or a spine fracture, don't receive the most effective medications to prevent future fractures. This is one area that, with simple steps, you can watch over for your health. It's as simple as a bone density test.

We recommend a DEXA test if one or more of the following situations apply to you:

- A fracture
- History of eating disorders
- Amenorrhea (loss of menstrual periods)
- Around the time of menopause
- Postmenopause
- Choosing not to take estrogen at menopause
- Taking medications for other health problems, listed on page 17, which can cause bone thinning, especially prednisone or other cortisone medication
- Taking bone-strengthening medications listed on page 111. (The bone density test is used to assess the effect of treatment.)
- Taking estrogen therapy for more than a few years
- Over age thirty with rheumatoid arthritis

- Men over age seventy, especially if they smoke, have lost height, take prednisone, or have chronic bronchitis, emphysema, or other medical problem (see section on men and osteoporosis on page 133).

Dr. Harris: "While there is much enthusiasm about the new bone density tests, it's important to note that this screening is not necessary for every young woman. Key factors such as age, lifestyle habits, and family history should be taken into consideration before you have this test done."

What to Expect

What are the preparations? You will be asked to lie down on a table or sit in a chair, but you won't have to undress (see photo). No pain or needles are involved.

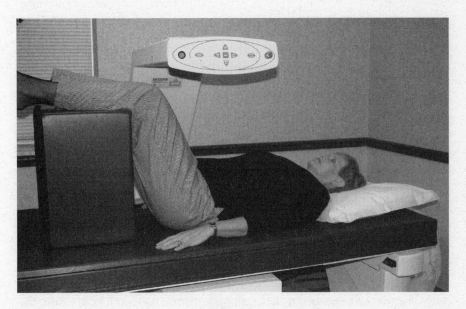

Figure 1.3

The DEXA bone density test

What happens during the scan? In the DEXA test, the machine passes over the hip and lumbar spine as you lie on the table. In the heel sonogram, you sit in a chair while the machine quickly measures the heel bone density. *Both bone density tests* are quick, taking only a few minutes to complete.

Is it safe? The DEXA test uses a very small amount of X ray to measure bone mass. Your exposure is much less than if you had a chest X ray or a mammogram or about as much as the amount of "natural" radiation one might receive on an airplane trip across the United States.

The heel sonogram uses sound waves, not X-ray beams, and has no long-term side effects or radiation.

How much does it cost? The DEXA scan costs about $125. Some doctor's offices offer heel sonogram tests that cost around $40, and you might even find free screening scans available at health fairs, shopping centers, and drugstores. Talk to your insurance provider to see if it is covered under your policy.

Who interprets the results? Once you get your test results, you should review these with your doctor. He or she can explain what your actual bone strength is and what options you have for prevention or treatment. Use the results as an early warning sign. It's never too early to prevent or reverse osteopenia and it's never too late to treat osteoporosis and fractures.

A Bone-Saving Fracture?

If you have already had a fracture, this may be a sign of significant or severe bone loss. It is very important that you have a bone density test, examine other risk factors, and decide with your doctor what prevention steps to take. Your signal fracture may be a blessing if it alerts you to a problem and leads you to take bone-saving action.

Bone density tests offer researchers insight into the devastation of bone loss. Using these tests, researchers have found that after a hip fracture, most patients lose even more bone and muscle, perhaps because of the forced loss of activity. Interestingly, one year after a hip fracture, some patients were found to have a 5 to 7 percent loss of bone density. In addition, the body's overall muscle mass after one year was down 5 to 9 percent. The loss of bone and muscle, along with the sudden loss of strength, may help explain why older patients experience serious problems after a hip fracture. This might also explain why so many never become independent or walk as well again.

Hip fractures also require surgery, and in patients who have a hip fracture from osteoporosis, about one-third have trouble with daily self-care and hygiene activities. Approximately one-fourth of hip fracture patients need long-term nursing home care, and there is a higher chance of death—over 20 percent the first year. Studies show that this number may increase to 50 percent or more for those over seventy-five.

Invest in Your Bones

There is a silver lining in the cloud of those sobering statistics. Using the newer methods of detecting bone loss, along with the latest prevention and medical treatments described in this book, the risk of osteopenia and fracture can be greatly reduced for most women. There is no need to suffer from a fracture—if you start investing in your bone health today.

To help determine the best course of action for you and your family, we wrote this book as the next best thing to consulting with you in person. As we explain to patients, *no single approach will solve the problem of bone loss*. What is called for is an individualized approach that considers all your specific risk factors. Once you've assessed your risk factors on page 15, follow the age-specific strategies in Steps 2 to 5 for ways to change those risks you can control. Ultimately, this will help you improve the strength of your bones and the quality of your life.

CHAPTER 2

Step 2: The Bone-Building Workout

There is no denying that medicine is changing at warp speed. While scientists continue to develop better ways to diagnose and treat bone loss, there remains a low-tech option for strengthening bones that won't ever change: *exercise*.

We know that it's hard to imagine how exercise can actually keep you from having a fracture or help you prevent a fall. After all, it seems logical that the more you move around, the greater the risk of injury or falling, which could result in a fracture.

But exercise *does* help prevent fractures—along with a host of other chronic diseases such as hypertension, cardiovascular disease, and diabetes. Not only does exercise keep bones strong, it strengthens your muscles which in turn support the joints, keeping them flexible and limber. If you've already experienced a fracture, exercise can shorten your recovery and even help to decrease the amount of pain you feel.

Exercise Tops the List

As discussed in Step 1, there are risk factors for bone loss and fractures you can change and risk factors over which you have no control. For example, you cannot change your gender, age, or family history. You can't avoid illnesses either—such as rheumatoid arthritis, asthma, thyroid disease, and inflammatory bowel disease, all risk factors for bone loss. Moreover, you cannot rewrite your personal health history. You may have avoided dairy products in your teen years or lived on a very low-calorie diet that was deficient in bone-boosting nutrients.

Nevertheless, there is one risk factor you can control—*you can change your exercise habits*, and here in Step 2 we will show you how easy it is to incorporate specific bone-building exercises in your daily routine.

If you are sedentary, we'll motivate you to *get up and get moving* in order to keep your bones strong. If you overexercise, we'll explain the importance of allowing for "rest" between workouts so you don't over-stress your body. Moreover, if you only do one type of exercise, such as marathon running, we'll explain why diversifying your workout is neces-sary to increase bone density and prevent fractures.

Starting today, you can make a commitment to get up and get moving with the Bone-Building Workout. In doing so, your bones will get stronger, your body will become more flexible, and your chances of suffer-ing with a painful, debilitating fracture will greatly diminish.

Before we explain how the Bone-Building Workout will keep your bones strong, let's look at a few of our patients who were diagnosed with bone loss at relatively young ages and how exercise helped them reverse this and regain control over their risk of fracture in later years:

Kate's Eating Disorder

> **Patient's Name:** Kate
> **Age:** 31
> **Diagnosis:** Osteopenia
> **Risk factors:** Eating disorders, irregular periods, low body fat,
>   family history

Thirty-one-year-old Kate had a lengthy history of low-calorie and dep-rivation dieting. "I was a perfectionist: the straight-A student, head cheer-leader and homecoming court," Kate said. "But when I left home to go away to college, I was overwhelmed with feelings of insecurity.

"I had difficulty adjusting to college life my freshman year. I ate to soothe my loneliness and gained more than twenty pounds. Instead of dealing with my changing body through additional exercise and proper food choices, I took control of my food intake. I ate enormous amounts of food [binge] late at night in the dorm, and then I'd throw up [purge] until my eyes were bloodshot. I did this bingeing-purging routine every night during my college years and finally was able to control my weight."

Kate said she continued her "secret" way of staying trim for more than a decade and was proud that she had less than 20 percent body fat and could wear a size 2. Nevertheless, as she approached thirty, her body began to change, and her periods became irregular. Her hair began to thin, her skin was dry and flaky, and the enamel on her teeth became worn. She finally came in for an evaluation after reading some magazine articles about eating disorders leading to osteopenia and fractures.

After reviewing Kate's medical and family history, we felt that a bone density test was warranted, especially since her mother was recently diagnosed with osteoporosis after suffering a fracture. Kate's DEXA bone density test showed osteopenia. We explained that osteopenia put her at a higher risk of fractures if she did not take precautions now and change those risk factors she could control.

Kate vowed to start the Bone-Building Workout, using a combination of daily weight bearing and strengthening exercises, a bone-boosting diet, and calcium supplements. We explained to Kate how exercise could help with her dieting obsession and allow her to maintain a normal weight without dangerously depriving herself of healthful nutrients. A revealing study from the University of Minnesota's Adolescent Health Program found that chronic dieters (those who dieted at least ten times a year) were

- 10 times more likely to vomit one or more times a week
- 8 times more likely to use ipecac to induce vomiting
- 7 times more likely to use laxatives to induce diarrhea
- 7 times more likely to use diuretics to dehydrate the body

Maintaining a normal weight would help Kate regulate her menstrual cycle, too. Researchers at West Virginia University found that women who exercised four days a week reduced their cravings for fatty foods as their body developed a taste for the right complex carbohydrates to fuel their workouts. Kate needed to learn how to eat right to stay healthy.

A year later, Kate's bone density test shows great improvement. She has stopped bingeing and purging and says she's never felt healthier.

Get the Facts on Eating Disorders

- By age five, most girls describe thin friends as more desirable than overweight ones.
- By age six, 40 percent have expressed a desire to be thinner.
- By age nine, nearly 50 percent have already embarked on their first restrictive diet.
- By age fifteen, one of eight girls is dieting at least ten times a year.
- By age sixteen, 45 percent are crash-dieting, 40 percent are fasting, and 15 percent are taking diet pills.
- By college, one in ten female college students exhibits disordered eating.

Liz's Exercise Compulsion

Patient's Name: Liz
Age: 29
Diagnosis: Osteopenia
Risk factors: Rigorous exercise, marathon runner, low body weight

Twenty-nine-year-old Liz, an intellectual property attorney, is another healthy young woman who found out she had osteopenia before having a fracture. Liz was a high school and college athlete—she ran track during high school and college, and played on a women's volleyball team that toured the United States doing exhibitions for other colleges. When Liz started law school, she didn't have time for recreational team sports, so she designed her own daily fitness program:

- A high-impact step aerobics class before school
- Thirty minutes on the Stairmaster during her lunch hour
- A three-mile run before dinner

When Liz joined a law practice in town, she continued her disciplined exercise regimen and started training for marathons on the weekends. Even though Liz ate a healthy diet, she had low body weight because of her rigorous exercise.

At one of the races, the sponsor offered free bone density tests for the athletes. Liz had a BMD test and got the shocking results that she had osteopenia and was at increased risk for fracture.

When Liz came to our clinic for an evaluation, we explained to her that mounting evidence concludes that too much physical activity can result in bone disorders. While moderate physical activity is crucial, we told Liz that overexercising may weaken bones because the hormonal imbalances from intense exercise lead to decreased bone mass.

In a quest to live longer and look younger, many women like Liz have become obsessed with rigorous training regimens. Ironically, in their overzealous pursuit of optimal fitness and low body fat, they put their bones at risk. For some healthy women, overexercise can result in loss of menstrual periods and osteopenia (see discussion of the Female Athlete Triad, page 3).

We gave Liz a copy of our Bone-Building Workout, which features a varied workout that allows for rest to prevent overexercise and burnout, along with information on specific nutrients and supplements to include in her diet to build bone strength. Liz took her diagnosis seriously and vowed to make some changes in her daily exercise routine.

As with Kate, the Bone-Building Workout allowed Liz to increase bone density at a time in her life when she still could. In doing so, both women reduced their risk of future fractures and put their minds at ease.

Signs and Symptoms of Eating Disorders

- Very low-calorie diet
- Extreme weight change
- Insomnia
- Constipation
- Skin rash or dry skin
- Loss of hair or nail quality
- Unusual eating habits, such as binge eating or skipping meals
- Hyperactivity and high interest in exercise
- Denial
- Changes in personality

Dr. Kim: "If distance running is your only form of exercise, start mixing it up with weight training and circuit training. A new study published in the February 2003 issue of the *British Journal of Sports Medicine* suggests that long-distance running may increase the risk of low bone density as the body begins to adapt to the exercise and it stops having a stimulatory effect on the bones. Now, don't stop running—running is an excellent form of exercise. Just add other exercises to this regimen to ensure strong bones."

Mona's Sedentary Job

Patient's Name: Mona
Age: 43
Diagnosis: Osteopenia
Risk factors: Sedentary lifestyle, lack of regular exercise, family history, cigarette smoking

When Mona's older sister fractured a bone and was diagnosed with osteoporosis, this forty-three-year-old technical writer was frightened. "Almost every older woman in our family has osteoporosis," Mona said. "My grandmother is in a nursing home with complications from a hip fracture. I just don't want to be a victim of this disease."

Mona's bone density test showed osteopenia. Even though she ate a nutritious diet and took calcium supplements, her sedentary job and lifestyle had to change. Also, Mona said that she had smoked at least a pack of cigarettes each day since college. We suggested that she immediately start the Bone-Building Workout, continue to follow a bone-boosting diet, and make a commitment to stop smoking.

At first, Mona embraced these key lifestyle changes. She made a pact with her husband to stop smoking and, with help from nicotine patches and an online support group, they quit. Mona also started the exercise program, scheduling time before work to walk two miles and do her strength training. However, after a few months, this early morning workout became difficult, especially on cold or rainy mornings. So, Mona "rewrote" her program, changing the workout to "weekends only." When she came back in for a bone density test, we were puzzled as to why she had no improvement, until she admitted that though she did the two-mile walks, she only did them on Saturday and Sunday.

Many of our patients, particularly women like Mona with full-time careers, opt to avoid exercise during the week and then use the weekend to catch up on exercise. Findings confirm that in order to build strong bones, you need regular, consistent movement. Comprehensive studies from the State University of New York show that postmenopausal women who walk one hour longer *per day* than other women have stronger, thicker bones in the hips—with bone mass comparable to women four years younger.

We explained to Mona the most dramatic demonstration of the interaction between activity and bone mass has come from studies of bed rest immobilization and the Sky Lab astronauts. Bone mineral loss of approximately 0.5 percent of the skeleton per month occurs with bed rest, with the majority of that loss apparently from the lower extremities.

Now that Mona has gone back to the Bone-Building Workout, her latest bone scan shows improvement in bone strength. She also feels more in control of her destiny, that she can prevent osteoporosis and fractures—no matter what her family history dictates.

Libby's Early Menopause

> **Patient's Name:** Libby
> **Age:** 46
> **Diagnosis:** Osteopenia
> **Risk factors:** Early surgical menopause with no estrogen replacement, spinal fractures

Libby's exercise program helped her to return to an active life. After having a surgical menopause at age forty, this forty-six-year-old accountant was bothered for several years by chronic pain in her middle and lower back. Libby excused the pain as the result of lifelong poor posture and did nothing to strengthen her back. One morning, Libby could not bend over to put on her shoes without excruciating pain in her middle back. She immediately made an appointment at the clinic.

When we first met Libby, she had severe pain in her middle and lower back and was afraid she'd have to stop work because the pain prevented sitting and standing for more than a few minutes at a time. X rays showed that Libby had several fractures in the vertebrae of the spine; a DEXA scan revealed osteopenia with a bone density of a postmenopausal woman.

Because Libby did not take estrogen replacement after her surgical menopause, she was at higher risk for osteoporosis and fractures. Unlike many forty-year-old women who are still menstruating and have the benefit of estrogen on their bones, Libby experienced rapid bone loss for the first few years after her surgery.

Libby immediately started medications to increase bone density and prevent future fractures. She also added bone-boosting foods to her diet and calcium supplements, and started the weight-bearing and strengthening exercises outlined in the *Bone-Building Program*. Over time, she slowly increased the exercises as her pain subsided, and within a few weeks, she was walking on her treadmill in the morning and riding bikes in the evenings with her teenage daughters. One year after starting the Bone-Building Workout, Libby's bone density had dramatically improved. She was determined to never suffer another fracture again.

For Libby, the Bone-Building Workout achieved two goals:

1. It strengthened her back muscles, and gave more support and flexibility to the spine and nearby soft tissues, resulting in much less pain.
2. It helped to increase the bone density in the spine, which was insurance against future fractures.

Never Too Late

For some women reading this book, regular exercise is already an important part of their health-conscious lifestyle. However, the reality is that many others completely ignore this discipline and unless they make a commitment could face painful, debilitating fractures down the road. No matter what your age or fitness level, it's never too late to get up and start walking—or dancing, jogging, playing tennis, climbing stairs, or any weight-bearing activity that keeps bones strong.

Focus on Two Types of Exercise

We teach our patients that two different types of exercise are necessary to keep bones strong and prevent osteopenia, osteoporosis, and fractures:

1. Weight-bearing exercise—including exercise that forces your body to resist gravity
2. Strength training or resistance exercise—including exercise that strengthens back muscles

Weight-Bearing Exercise

Weight-bearing exercises, including walking, aerobics, dancing, climbing stairs, jogging, racquet sports, running, yoga, tai chi, Pilates, and water aerobics, are all crucial to increasing bone mass—no matter what your age. (Swimming is an excellent cardiovascular and back exercise, but it is not weight-bearing.)

How does it work? Weight-bearing exercise stimulates cells in the body that make new bone. By doing these exercises daily, you can encourage your body to build bone and delay or reverse osteopenia, osteoporosis, and fractures. When you add resistance or strength training exercises to this regimen, you will become more flexible and reduce the likelihood of falling—the number one risk factor for hip fracture (see page 6). We believe this is a very small price to pay to live stronger and fracture-free.

How much is enough? Exercise does not have to be excessive or strenuous to stop or reverse bone loss. In a study involving more than eight hundred older adults, which was published in the *American Journal of Clinical Nutrition*, researchers found that those who walked the equivalent of at least 20 to 30 minutes per day had significantly denser bones than inactive adults of the same age. Many other studies have made similar conclusions—weight-bearing exercise, such as walking, can stimulate bone in young, perimenopausal, postmenopausal, and elderly women.

Gardening for Your Health

If walking on a treadmill bores you and you don't want to join a fitness center, try gardening to reduce your risk of osteopenia and fractures. A study published in the May 2003 issue of the *National Women's Health Report* confirms that gardening may even be better than walking for reducing the risk of osteoporosis.

In the study, researchers reviewed data for 3,310 women aged fifty and older who were part of the Third National Health and Nutrition Examination Survey (NHANES III). They confirm that only weight training is better than yard work as an activity associated with reducing the risk of bone loss and fractures.

If you garden, you know how much physical effort is involved. However, as researchers substantiate, gardening also gives pleasure so that people are likely to stay with it.

2,000 Steps to Lovely Bones

Some walkers get a pedometer to measure steps or distance. Studies show that 2,000 steps translate to roughly 1 mile. Start with 250 steps (quarter-mile) and make your next goal 500 steps. Continue to increase the step count until you reach an optimal goal of 2,000 steps (1 mile) or more each exercise session.

While there are no definitive studies pinpointing the optimal amount of weight-bearing exercise, we recommend that patients aim for 30 to 45 minutes at least five days a week. Some research findings show that for postmenopausal women, a 60-minute workout performed three times a week can stop bone loss. In a study of 266 women—average age fifty five, average weight 155—published in the August 2003 issue of the journal *Osteoporosis International*, researchers assigned half of the participants to the exercise regimen plus a calcium supplement and half to just calcium alone. After one year, those women in the exercise group had better bone mineral density than the nonexercisers.

If you are new to exercise and have been sedentary for a while, go slowly. Start by walking only a few minutes, gradually building up to your personal goal of 30 to 45 minutes, five days a week. The rule should be that when you finish walking, you should have no pain or discomfort. Then gradually increase the distance.

How do you know it's working? Just as you don't see bone loss over the years, you cannot tell when your bones respond to exercise. Still, when you land on your feet during a walk or run, specific chemical messengers signal your leg bones to be ready to handle that weight and impact again.

Strength Training (Resistance Exercise)

Strength training (or resistance exercise) helps to reduce the risk for bone loss by causing the muscles to pull on the bone, resulting in in-creased bone strength. Examples of low-intensity resistance include using an elastic resistance band, your own weight as resistance, lifting canned goods, or lifting bags of groceries or a baby. Moderate-intensity resistance includes a medium-intensity exercise band, free weights, ankle and wrist weights, weight machines, or your own body weight. High-intensity exer-cises include using heavier free weights (barbells) or weight machines.

Weight-training equipment that allows you to exercise standing up in a "weight-bearing position" may help you build bone more effectively than weight training in a sitting position.

Study after study reinforces the beneficial effects of strength training, including increased bone mass, muscular strength, power, dynamic balance, and functional independence. Strength training is also important in the development and maintenance of fat-free mass (FFM) and in improving and maintaining muscular strength. In findings published in the January 2003 issue of *Medicine and Science in Sports and Exercise*, researchers confirmed a significant progressive relationship between total weight lifted and an increase in bone density in a study of postmenopausal women who ingested ample calcium. For women who opt not to use hormone replacement therapy, strength training can partially substitute for the bone-stimulating effects of estrogen.

Strength training is also excellent for building muscle, especially in the back. When these muscles become stronger, the bone density in the spine increases, helping to add strength to the entire skeleton. Medical research shows that strength training is key to preventing sarcopenia, the age-related loss of muscle mass that is associated with reduced muscle strength and reduced endurance. A sedentary lifestyle and menopause both accelerate the process of sarcopenia. You can prevent sarcopenia with resistance training, and consistent exercise may even reverse it.

Dr. Laura: "Balancing my roles as wife, mother, and doctor, I know the importance of being strong. Strength training does help. Not only does the resistance workout help prevent bone loss and fractures, but regular workouts improve posture and confidence and can improve a woman's body image even better than aerobics. Strength training puts women in touch with their bodies and helps us see them as allies. As with starting any exercise program, you should discuss this with your doctor first."

How does it work? Unlike aerobic exercise, which is low resistance, rhythmic, and uses multiple muscle groups at the same time, strength training uses some form of tension or resistance on core muscle groups.

How much is enough? Aim for two or three times a week as you start strengthening exercises, and then increase if you are able. Always allow for at least 24 hours between sessions for your body to rest. Over time, your goal should be to increase the duration of each session. Alternate upper-body and lower-body routines.

Initially, use low resistance—two to five pounds. It's important to concentrate on form and technique rather than the amount of weight. Once you find a comfortable weight, stay with it for one to two sets of ten repetitions per body part, taking one to three minutes between sets to ensure a good quality workout.

Some newer studies show bone responds better to higher loads of low frequency than to frequent repetitions of low loads (weights). In other words, lifting 25 pounds ten times may be more effective in stimulating bone than lifting 5 pounds fifty times. In medical studies of bone density, findings show that swimmers had the lowest bone density among athletes and Olympic weight-lifters had the highest. We recommend starting with lower weight that you can use comfortably without injury or pain.

If you choose to use the strengthening and range-of-motion exercises in chapter 8 of this book, start with only one or two of each exercise, so that you do not overextend underused muscles and joints. Gradually increase the number of repetitions per set and the number of sessions per week.

How do you know it's working? Most of our patients say they feel stronger after just a few weeks of doing strength-training sessions. In a study published in the journal *Medicine and Science in Sports and Exercise*, researchers conclude that resistance training for three to six months can improve muscular strength and endurance by 25 to 100 percent—depending on the workout and the woman's initial level of strength. You may also notice that your muscle tone is firm or that you've lost a few pounds. (Weight training builds muscle and muscle burns fat, resulting in weight loss for most women.)

Dr. Kim: "Research shows that muscle weakness in the back and legs is a major contributor to falls. When you add in other factors such as a sedentary lifestyle, diminished vision, and certain medications, it becomes apparent why falls are more frequent as we age. We also know that frequent falls can result in increased risk of fracture, immobility, and even death. The good news is that with exercise and stronger muscles a person's ability to stand and walk improves."

Dr. Laura: "If you experience any pain during the Bone-Building Workout, stop the exercise. Some muscle fatigue is to be expected during weight-bearing or strength-training exercise. However, if you feel acute or sharp stabbing pain, this is a warning that you are straining too hard or performing the exercise incorrectly. If this happens, talk to your doctor or a physical therapist about proper exercise form. As with starting any exercise program, you should discuss this with your doctor first."

Exercise Benefits Outweigh the Risks

No matter what your age or fitness level, we believe that every woman can exercise in some way. The benefits far outweigh the risks. Even after a fracture in the spine, you will soon be able to walk, and then gradually begin gentle exercises. A physical therapist can be a great help at this time by showing you the proper way to exercise safely.

Tai Chi Can Prevent Falls

Tai chi is an exercise that originated in China. Using slow, graceful movements, you will work all parts of the body while standing (weight-bearing). Because of the slow movements, tai chi helps to improve balance and flexibility. Tai chi works for all ages.

A study from Emory University published in 1996 in the *Journal of the American Medical Association* evaluated various types of exercise and reported that tai chi significantly decreased the risk of falls when compared to other activities. Other findings presented at the annual meeting of the American College of Rheumatology (December 2001) by researchers from Korea reported similar results. These scientists found that tai chi may help some with arthritis. At the end of the two-week study, women in the tai chi group reported less pain, fewer difficulties with daily activities, improved balance, and greater abdominal muscle strength. In yet another comprehensive study, reported in the *Townsend Letter for Doctors* (July 2000), researchers showed that by doing tai chi for one hour a week for two months, there was a significant improvement in four out of five measures of balance.

Call your local fitness center for instruction in this ancient discipline or get a tai chi demonstration video at your local library or bookstore.

Body Benefits

Aside from building bone and helping to prevent falls, exercise gives other benefits to your body. For example, regular exercise reduces the amount of adrenaline circulating in the body, which relaxes blood vessels and results in a slower pulse rate and lower blood pressure. Aerobic activity such as walking also helps to raise your HDL (good) cholesterol and lower your LDL (bad) cholesterol and triglycerides. Studies show that just three hours of walking each week (about a half hour each day) can reduce a woman's risk of heart attack by 35 percent.

A regular exercise routine also reduces a woman's risk of colon and breast cancer. In a 2001 study published in the journal *Medicine and Science in Sports and Exercise*, researchers state that the breast cancer benefit is especially pronounced in perimenopausal women under the age of forty-five.

Mind and Spirit Benefits

There are still more benefits of exercise for women. Regular exercise produces alpha waves in the brain that are tied to feelings of serenity. It reduces anxiety and stress and might improve mood in those with depression. Exercise also releases endorphins, which are brain chemicals that are natural mood elevators. Almost all of my patients who exercise regularly experience improved sleep.

---

10 Exercise Benefits

1. Keeps muscles strong and joints limber.
2. Builds endurance and strengthens the cardiovascular system.
3. Boosts bone density to prevent fractures.
4. Sharpens reaction time and helps decrease risk of falls. Exercise boosts oxygen to the brain, which is then sent to your muscles.
5. Lowers blood pressure and heart rate.
6. Improves mood and sleep.
7. Burns fat and helps to maintain a normal weight.
8. Helps reduce the risk of diabetes mellitus.
9. Relieves tension and helps keep you alert.
10. Improves self-image.

It's Never Too Late

Forty-six-year-old Carmen is an avid walker. She walks to the grocery store, to her part-time job at a local elementary school, to visit with friends and family, and even to our clinic more than two miles from her home. "Not only do I enjoy walking, but it helps me stay fit and strong."

She wasn't always so gung-ho. Two years ago, she bent over to pick up one of the kindergarten students at school and fractured a vertebra in her spine. A bone density test showed osteopenia. After weeks of excruciating pain, Carmen made up her mind that this would never happen to her again. We talked about the importance of regular weight-bearing exercise, along with dietary changes, to build strong bones. Because Carmen had a

Avoid Overtraining

Now, while we want you to get up and get moving, we don't want you to overtrain. In fact, most exercise physiologists say that rest is the second half of any workout. Athletes have learned that peak performance comes from scheduling periods of rest between their training sessions. Many coaches and athletes use the terms "rest" and "recovery" interchangeably, but rest actually refers to doing nothing, and recovery is the period immediately following a workout when your body adjusts to the exercise before it returns to its resting state.

By resting, you allow the body a chance to adjust to the stress put upon it by walking, running, dancing, weight training, or other activities. When you slowly increase the frequency of your workouts, their length or intensity, and then you rest for a certain time, your body becomes stronger and fit. When you weight train, even with light weights, it is best to lift weights two or three times a week with 24 to 36 hours of rest between sessions.

Overtraining increases the likelihood of injury, sickness, and fatigue. While regular, consistent exercise boosts your immune system, excessive exercise (to the point of exhaustion) or overtraining can negatively affect it. When you overtrain, your body dumps emergency hormones like adrenaline and cortisol into the bloodstream. These hormones help you cope with the physical stress but can also increase your likelihood of sickness and disease. Overexercising can also cause fatigue, insomnia, and lack of interest in sex. If you want to exercise frequently, alternate between light and heavy training days.

surgical menopause in her late thirties and had not taken hormone replacement therapy, we started her on Actonel (risedronate, discussed on page 109), to increase bone mass and lower her risk of fractures.

Today Carmen's bones are measurably stronger. Not only has walking improved her bone strength, she also feels less stress, her mood is more positive, and she can keep up with her twenty-two active kindergarten students.

You may be in your 30s, 40s, or 50s and wonder how you can start a regular exercise program. Well, we have hundreds of older patients—in their 60s, 70s, 80s, and even 90s who exercise every day without fail. Our patients say that when they exercise they feel better. So what are you waiting for?

Make the Commitment

Starting today, we want you to make a commitment to build better bones, avoid fractures, and live a stronger, healthier life. Just as you set personal or career goals, you must also set goals for your Bone-Building Workout. For instance, planning time for exercise is crucial. Many women say that early morning is the best time to exercise if you want to stick with it. (As one patient shared, "Exercising early in the morning keeps me from thinking of one hundred reasons not to exercise throughout the day! The longer I wait to exercise, the more I talk myself out of doing it at all.") Whatever time you choose, try to stay with this if possible. Some examples of goals include:

- I will stay with the workout for at least three months.
- I will block time in my daily routine for my workout.
- I will not let other commitments or people stop me from this workout time.
- I will think positive and healing thoughts about exercise before I work out.
- I will focus on the fact that the workout will help me stay strong and healthy the rest of my life.

According to a report by the Centers for Disease Control and Prevention (CDC), only about one in five American adults takes on a high level of physical activity, and one in four engages in little or no regular physical activity. If you fall into the inactive category with little or no regular physical exercise, vow to change this sedentary habit. Starting today, set the goals of beginning slowly and allowing ample time to get used to the increased activity.

Precautions If You've Had a Fracture

If you have had a recent fracture, begin your exercise program only when your doctor gives approval. An easy start would be to walk across your living room several times a day. Then each day slowly increase the duration of your workout. Walk through your house for five, then ten minutes at a time. If you have no pain or other difficulty walking, consider walking outdoors, every other day for a week or two.

As you adjust to this walk, add five, then ten minutes to each session. You can do this twice a day or every day until you can build your strength and endurance to walk a total of thirty to forty minutes, three or four times each week or more often. Increasing slowly is better than overexercising and risking injury.

Once you make a commitment to your daily exercise program, stick with it. Using a calendar, check off the days that you exercise, recording the length of each workout session and the distance you covered. Remember, your bones did not weaken overnight; it will take time to build strength.

Consult with a Physical Therapist

Beginning your program with the help and instruction of a physical therapist may be beneficial. This therapist can tell you if you are doing the exercises correctly so that you get the maximum benefit. The therapist can also instruct you with the proper use of moist heat, hot packs, and other helpful treatments if you experience pain or stiffness during your regimen.

Rate Your Level of Activity

Rating	Type of Activity
Inactivity	Using the computer, watching television
No impact	Swimming
Low impact	Pleasure cycling, a stroll through the park
Moderate impact	Dancing, walking 3 mph
High impact	Step aerobics, walking 4 mph, jogging

Daily Living Activities Do Count

For those who want to run the other way when someone mentions starting an exercise program, here's some good news: you don't have to go to a fitness center in order to keep bones strong. Exercise can be any type of physical movement, including household or daily activities such as mopping or vacuuming floors, washing windows, raking your yard, or carrying bags of groceries into your home.

If you are too busy to plan at least 30 minutes of weight-bearing or strengthening exercises each day, try increasing your daily activity level instead. Make sure the activities are weight-bearing and strengthening to get the full bone-boosting benefit. For example, you can include anything from active housework and gardening to using the stairs instead of the elevator, to walking your dog in the evening after work. If you are going shopping, park at the back of the lot and walk the extra distance. Instead of letting someone help you with your groceries, lift the bags yourself and count this as part of your strengthening program. If you see trash on the ground, bend over and pick it up. Movements like this will keep you flexible and in shape no matter what your age.

Train your mind to think—*more activity instead of less*. Then make it your goal to accumulate at least 30 minutes of activity each day.

Examples of Bone-Building Daily Activities

- Dusting (actively)
- Gardening
- Mowing the lawn
- Playing actively with children or grandchildren
- Pushing a stroller
- Raking leaves
- Running
- Stair walking
- Walking the dog
- Washing and waxing a car
- Washing windows or floors

Dr. Laura: "My grandmother has never been to a fitness center or gym. Jewel is nevertheless a youthful, energetic, and meticulous housekeeper, and does all her home and yard maintenance. If she's not making beds, mopping, or vacuuming, she's outside planting rosebushes, washing windows, or raking her large lawn. Jewel thinks nothing of bringing her own groceries in from the car or carrying out heavy garbage cans to the curb. It's not surprising that she's also in perfect health and has very strong bones. My grandmother is confirmation to me that daily household and living activities can keep bones strong and help you to stay in good physical shape."

Your Bone-Building Workout

In our clinic, we've found that the "one size fits all" approach to exercise simply does not work. One of the more important concepts in the effective prescription of exercise for any age group is to design the exercise program specifically for the individual. With this Bone-Building Workout, you can select the exercises and activities you most enjoy. Studies show that in the prevention of osteoporosis, gains in skeletal mineral content made earlier in life may not be sustained later in life. So, for exercise to be effective it must be ongoing. Exercise isn't a quick fix or short-term remedy.

Add Music to Your Exercise Regimen

Researchers in the Department of Physical Therapy at Springfield College in Massachusetts found that people who exercise to music will stay with it longer than if they work out in silence. Men and women riding stationary bikes rode from 25 to 29 percent longer listening to their favorite tunes.

Before You Begin

Check with your doctor if you are over forty years old or if you have not exercised for a while. Also check with your doctor if you have risk factors for cardiovascular disease such as smoking, high blood pressure, high total cholesterol, diabetes, obesity, or a sedentary lifestyle. If you are experiencing occasional or frequent chest pains, feel faint or dizzy, or are taking prescription medication such as treatment for hypertension, make sure your doctor monitors your exercise and your progress.

The Bone-Building Workout

Weight-bearing Exercise + Resistance Training =
Strong Bones and No Fractures

Get Ready to Work Out
5 Minutes before Exercise
To begin your exercise program, walk in place, march, or walk up and down stairs to get your blood flowing and prepare your body for the workout.

Weight-Bearing Activities
Weight-bearing exercises help you to move your body against gravity. Depending on your level of fitness, choose an exercise you love from the following weight-bearing activities, which are proven to strengthen bone.

We've found that moderate physical activity is a level of exercise most healthy women can achieve and it will promote bone strength when combined with a diet high in calcium and other bone-boosting nutrients.

Low Intensity	Moderate Intensity	High Intensity
Ballroom dancing (light)	Aerobics (low-impact)	Aerobics (high-impact)
Golf (with cart)	Badminton	Basketball
Tai chi	Ballroom dancing (fast)	Dancing (fast)
Water aerobics (slow tempo)	Cycling (leisure)	Hiking
Yoga	Golf (carry clubs)	Jogging
	Mall walking (3–4 mph)	Jumping rope
	Stair climbing	Rollerblading
	Tae kwon do	Soccer
	Tennis (doubles)	Tennis (singles)
	Walking, brisk	
	Water aerobics (moderate tempo)	

Cooldown
5 Minutes after Exercise
Follow the stretching exercises on page 187 as you end your weight-bearing exercise routine. Gently do the stretches, holding each one 20 seconds without bouncing.

Strength-Training Exercises
Alternate strength-training or resistance workouts with weight-bearing workouts two or three times a week. Be sure to allow for a rest day in-between workouts. Your strength-training workout should include:

- 8 to 10 exercises for the major muscle groups, using the exercises explained on page 35
- 1 to 2 sets of each exercise with 10 to 15 repetitions per set

If you are using free weights or weight machines at a local fitness center, then slowly increase the weight after you can comfortably perform fifteen repetitions. A trainer or assistant can be of great help as you begin your exercise program.

Yoga for Better Bones

Many of our patients are avid proponents of yoga, an ancient Indian practice, taking group classes at the local Y or at exercise facilities in the area. It's estimated that more than 20 million Americans now practice yoga. The various slow-motion postures and deep-breathing exercises help to integrate the body, breath, and mind, and can help strengthen muscles, as well as alleviate emotional stress.

Bone-Building Homework

As you increase in strength and endurance, try the following weight-bearing/resistance combination exercises to get an extra bone-boosting benefit. We've found these to be excellent exercises especially when you don't have time to go to the gym or fitness center:

- Walk the dog wearing strap-on ankle or wrist weights.
- Clean house wearing strap-on ankle or wrist weights.
- Garden or do yard work wearing strap-on ankle weights.
- Use an older style lawn mower that you must push and pull.
- Push a baby stroller wearing strap-on ankle weights.
- Do low-impact aerobics or step aerobics with strap-on ankle or wrist weights.
- Do step aerobics class with strap-on ankle or wrist weights.
- Use elastic resistance bands while watching television or a video.

Age-Specific Bone-Building Recommendations

20s to 30s

While most of your bone mass is achieved by the time you are in your 20s, increases in bone density have been observed throughout the third decade of life. Studies show that just a moderate increase in weight-bearing exercise and strength training can build bone. Even small improvements in bone mass in young to middle adulthood may result in quite significant reductions in risk for osteoporotic fractures after menopause. Start your Bone-Building Workout now—before perimenopause and the decline of bone-boosting estrogen occur. This is a great time to start a lifelong weight-bearing and strengthening program.

Recommendations

- **5 days a week:** Select a workout activity from the list on page 45. If you work full-time and are unable to exercise outdoors, we recommend an indoor treadmill, stair machine, or a cross-trainer, which provides both aerobic and resistance training. Start with 30 minutes initially and increase in 5-minute increments, as you are able. Your goal is to build to 45 minutes (or more) of weight-bearing exercise, five days a week.
- **Variations**:
  - Carry free weights in hands, walk with strap-on ankle weights, or push a stroller while walking.
  - Use hand-iron gloves (weighted gloves of 1 to 3 pounds for each hand). These gloves are safer for the wrists than hand weights and they free up your hands.
  - If you live near the beach, substitute power walking in sand for one of your weight-bearing workouts each week.
- **2–3 days a week:** Start strengthening exercises, as discussed on page 35, for 15 minutes. Use weights or resistance machines with moderate resistance. Increase to 20 minutes as you're able. Allow 24 hours for the body to rest between workouts.
- **3 days a week:** Add swimming to strengthen back muscles. Strong back muscles support the spine and encourage good posture.

A weekly workout schedule might look something like this:

Monday	40-minute walk with friends
Tuesday	15 minutes of resistance machines at Y; 30-minute freestyle swim
Wednesday	45-minute morning walk pushing baby stroller
Thursday	15 minutes of resistance machines at Y; water aerobics class; 15 minutes freestyle swim
Friday	1 hour dancing at club; household chores
Saturday	15 minutes free weights and isometrics at home; household and gardening activities (3 hours)
Sunday	45-minute bike ride in the park

40s

Many women become more sedentary as children grow up and household responsibilities lessen. At this age, you may have gone back to work full-time and relish being able to sit down and catch your breath instead of chasing little ones across the playground. The problem is that this is the age, before menopause, when women need to stay even more focused on a regular weight-bearing and strengthening exercise program in order to build as much bone as possible. Planning periods of physical activity throughout the day may be necessary from midlife on as your activity levels might otherwise diminish significantly. This is the time to begin a program that can make a difference in your bones and your overall health.

If you now have a sedentary lifestyle, you may benefit the most from increased exercise. Some findings consistently report that when sedentary adults start a regular exercise program, their bones reap the benefits.

Recommendations

- **5 days a week:** Choose a workout activity from the list on page 45. Start with 25 minutes daily and increase in 5-minute increments, as you are able. Build to 40 minutes (or more) of weight-bearing exercise, five days a week. If you use a treadmill, increase the incline or use ankle weights to increase the intensity of your workouts as needed.
- **2–3 days a week:** Start strengthening exercises, as discussed on page 35, for 10 minutes. Start with low-intensity free weights or

resistance machines. Increase to 20 minutes. Allow 24 hours for the body to rest between workouts.

- **2 days a week:** Add swimming to strengthen back muscles. Strong back muscles support the spine. Add resistance such as a kickboard to help strengthen muscles.
- **Other:**
  - Take a yoga or tai chi class to increase flexibility.
  - Include other daily activities such as gardening and walking stairs at work to boost your Bone-Building Workout.

A weekly workout schedule might look like this:

Monday	25-minute walk on indoor treadmill
Tuesday	10 minutes strengthening exercises using free weights; 1 hour gardening
Wednesday	30-minute walk at the mall with friends
Thursday	15 minutes of resistance machines at Y; tai chi class
Friday	30-minute walk during lunch hour; household chores (1 hour)
Saturday	15 minutes resistance machines at Y; family swim for 45 minutes
Sunday	2 hours gardening

50s and 60s

The three to five years following menopause are the "danger zone" when it comes to bone health because of the rapid withdrawal of estrogen. During this time, you can lose from 10 to 15 percent of your bone mass. Still, as with other age groups, women who stay physically active with a regular weight-bearing and resistance exercise program fare better than women who ignore exercise and have a sedentary lifestyle.

Even though you might feel like relaxing more at this life stage (and you've probably earned it!), it's essential to incorporate weight-bearing exercise, as well as strength training into your daily routine. Over a period of time, strength training will not only prevent bone loss, it can also help you to build stronger muscles, stay at a normal weight, and improve your overall health.

A comprehensive study published in the January 2003 issue of the journal *Medicine and Science in Sports and Exercise* reinforces the positive link between muscle-strengthening and osteoporosis prevention in women. The study also indicates a significant, progressive relationship between total weight lifted by postmenopausal women with adequate calcium and an increase in bone density.

In this particular study, researchers took bone density tests before and after each exercise period and compared these. The impact of each exercise on each measurement site was also assessed. The most significant increase in BMD was found in the hip site known as the *femur trochanter*, one of the most important weight-bearing structures in the body. The exercise found to have the most impact on this bone density increase was weighted squats, while weighted marching seemed to positively impact total body BMD most.

Another study, published in the November 2002 *Journal of the American Medical Association*, reveals that walking substantially reduces the risk of hip fracture. In this analysis of data from the United States Nurses' Health Study, researchers confirm that walking four hours per week reduces the risk of hip fracture in healthy postmenopausal women by 41 percent compared to walking less than one hour a week or not at all. Not only is walking safe and fun to do with family or friends, it is thought to increase hip bone density.

Recommendations

- **5 days a week:** Choose a workout activity from the list on page 45. We recommend walking to our patients, as there is no special equipment required and you can go at your own pace. Start with 20 minutes daily and increase in 5-minute increments, as you are able. Your goal is to build to 35 minutes (or more) of weight-bearing exercise, five days a week.
- **2–3 days a week:** Start strengthening exercises, as discussed on page 35, for 10 minutes. Use low intensity free weights or resistance machines. Increase to 20 minutes. Allow 24 to 36 hours for the body to rest between workouts.
- **2 days a week:** Add swimming to strengthen back muscles.
- **Other:**
  - Join an aquatics class at your local Y. Water aerobics can help to strengthen muscles yet are easy on aging joints.
  - Include other daily activities such as gardening and walking stairs at work to boost your Bone-Building Workout.

A weekly workout schedule might look like this:

Monday	20 minutes on treadmill (2 sets of 10 minutes each); gardening
Tuesday	10 minutes using free weights; 10 minutes of range of motion exercises (from chapter 8)
Wednesday	20 minutes on treadmill; 30-minute swim at club
Thursday	15 minutes at resistance machines; yoga class at Y
Friday	30 minutes on treadmill (3 sets of 10 minutes each); vacuuming and mopping
Saturday	Swim at club with family (1 hour); gardening and household chores
Sunday	Hike with family in local park (1 hour)

70 and over

In the past decade, we've seen a large increase in the number of women in their 80s and 90s who are physically active, but, sadly, more than half of women in this age group engage in no regular physical activity. In many cases, an exercise program can begin slowly and safely with excellent results.

Muscle weakness is associated with slow gait, slow chair rise, and dependence in Activities of Daily Living (ADLs). Resistance or strength training can help to increase strength, even with the frail elderly. Strength training is becoming quite common for many elderly people as they use their muscles repeatedly against a mobile, weighted resistance. Strength training can be performed using isometrics (see page 191), free weights, elastic bands, or resistive machines. A particular study conducted at the University of Colorado at Boulder looked at eleven men and women aged seventy to ninety-two. These elderly people—average age eighty—spent six months in an exercise program that included weight lifting. Under close supervision, they used weights that for them were heavy (the amount of weight varied per person). By the end of the study, all the participants showed considerable gains in balance and strength—some women more than doubled their strength in certain areas.

Recommendations

- **Daily:** Talk to your doctor about your specific health needs and exercise capability. Then get started by walking around a room, your home or apartment. Get up frequently instead of being sedentary. Increase the duration of your exercise sessions and the variety of your physical activity—as you are able to do so safely and comfortably.

- **Daily:** Stay active with daily living activities. Refer to our books *Pain-Free Arthritis* (Owl) and *The Pain-Free Back* (Owl) for helpful tips on pain-free gardening, travel, and other activities if you have arthritis or back pain.
- **2 days a week:** Enroll in a seniors' exercise or aquatics class at the local Y or arthritis foundation in your town.

A weekly workout schedule might look like this:

Monday	Water aerobics and stretching at Y (20 minutes)
Tuesday	Mall walk with neighbors (20 minutes); daily living activities
Wednesday	10-minute walk on treadmill; gardening (1 hour)
Thursday	Grocery shopping and kitchen clean-up (2 hours)
Friday	10-minute walk on treadmill; household chores
Saturday	Swim with grandchildren at club (30 minutes); gardening (1 hour)
Sunday	Neighborhood walk with friends (20 minutes); daily living activities

CHAPTER 3

Step 3: Feed Your Bones

At forty-three, Allison was a successful school administrator. She was a single mom and frequently participated in fund-raising walks for charity. Although Allison was underweight, smoked, and had avoided milk most of her life because of dairy allergies, she was a muscular, regular exerciser and never thought of herself as a candidate for early bone loss—until the day she tripped on her son's skateboard and fractured both her ankle and wrist.

After seeking treatment at a nearby emergency room, Allison came to our clinic for a bone density test. The result? A T score of -2.5, indicating the bone density of a woman years older. We talked with Allison about her personal and family medical history and found out that her grandmother and mother had bone loss with fractures. After reviewing the 12 risk factors on page 15, Allison understood that the probability for more fractures was extremely high, even for a perimenopausal woman in her early forties.

To look at Allison, you certainly would not target her as a candidate for early bone loss, especially if you saw her competing against women ten to twenty years younger in a 5K race. However, Allison and millions of other unsuspecting young and middle-aged women do have undiagnosed osteopenia and are headed for early painful fractures. Let's look at common dietary threads that weave many of these patients together:

Erin's Eating Disorders and Avoidance of Dairy Products

When Erin's menstrual periods stopped suddenly at age thirty-five, her gynecologist referred her to our clinic for a bone density test. In a desperate effort to stay slim, this young woman had suffered with eating disorders (binge eating and vomiting) since her freshman year in college and avoided dairy products for fear of gaining weight. At 5'4", Erin had a petite frame and weighed 105 pounds. We know that low body weight, with low percent body fat, can cause the body to end the production of estrogen, which probably led to Erin's amenorrhea (absent menstrual periods). Her grandmother and mother were both petite and had painful fractures at a young age.

Kaitlyn's Very Low-Calorie Diet

Twenty-two-year-old Kaitlyn was referred to our clinic after an ankle fracture and undergoing a bone density test offered by the student health center at her university. The test revealed that this young athlete had low bone mass and was at increased risk of more fractures. An avid exerciser, Kaitlyn played on the university's volleyball team and stayed on a very low-fat diet (less than 10 percent fat calories) to control her weight. (Very low-fat diets can result in low energy and performance and deficiencies in iron, zinc, magnesium, calcium, and other key nutrients.) Because of rigorous training, Kaitlyn had not had a menstrual period in more than a year (see Understanding the Female Athlete Triad, page 3). Her mother, age forty-four, was recently diagnosed with osteoporosis with fracture.

Jen's Avoidance of Dairy and History of Weight Cycling

Forty-four-year-old Jen, a successful intellectual property attorney, had a lengthy history of weight cycling or yo-yo dieting (repeated weight loss and weight gain, a common pattern among women who are trying to control obesity). Jen was overweight as a child so her pediatrician put her on a restricted low-calorie diet. She grew up avoiding dairy products and still despised the taste of low-fat milk, yogurt, and cheese. This avoidance of high-calcium dairy products continued through adulthood. Today, Jen's bone density test is like that of a much older woman.

Eating Disorders and Bone Loss

It is no news that America is a nation obsessed with being thin. We starve our bodies and sweat through grueling workouts in hopes of achieving that picture-perfect body. To stay slim, we cut back on calories, fats, and carbs and even harbor eating disorders and exercise obsessions.

What happens when we neglect our personal nutritional needs in pursuit of the perfect body? The bone health crisis American women face today is serious. Especially with women having *one out of two chances of fracturing a bone*—thin bones is one time when *thin is not attractive!*

When we examine severely underweight teenagers or young women who have fractures, we immediately suspect the possibility of an eating disorder. According to the American Academy of Child and Adolescent Psychiatry, anorexia nervosa and bulimia nervosa are eating disorders that are increasing among teens and kids, especially among young women. The American Anorexia/Bulimia Association estimates that 1 percent of teenage girls in the United States develop anorexia nervosa and up to 10 percent of those may die as a result. Approximately 5 percent of college women in the United States have bulimia.

What is it? An eating disorder is characterized by a morbid fear of weight gain that leads to severe restriction of food intake, resulting in extreme weight loss or starvation. Anorexia nervosa is self-starvation, a refusal to sustain a minimally normal body weight. With anorexia nervosa, a person literally starves herself to be thin and experiences excessive weight loss that can lead to serious illness or even death.

Bulimia nervosa involves repeated episodes of binge eating, followed by purging (vomiting or using laxatives). Someone with bulimia might experience fluctuations in weight yet these are not as extreme as with anorexia. Both anorexia and bulimia often occur along with compulsive exercise.

Who is at risk? Although eating disorders can occur in midlife, they are more common for people in their teens and 20s. In fact, 90 percent of children and teens with eating disorders are girls. Some reports suggest that media images promoting too-thin female ideals also promote eating disorders.

Those with eating disorders are often introverted, perfectionists, and high achievers in school. Various types of emotional stress or even depression may lead to problems in someone's relationship with food. Body-image distortions are primarily associated with anorexia. For example, despite dramatic weight loss, an anorectic may still see herself as getting increasingly fatter.

What price do we pay in terms of bone health? Studies suggest that osteopenia is increasingly common in those with eating disorders. Up to two-thirds of teens with anorexia have bone density values *significantly* below the norm. We know that girls with anorexia are less likely to achieve a peak bone density, which puts them at high risk for osteopenia and fracture throughout life. The low body weight results in the body ending the production of estrogen, which can contribute to amenorrhea (absent menstrual periods). Low estrogen levels lead to considerable losses in bone density. At our clinic, we've had patients with anorexia in their twenties who have had fractures from bone thinning.

Your Bone-Building Food Plan

"So, what foods do I eat to prevent osteopenia? I read a revealing magazine article that said dairy products might actually increase the risk of bone loss." Carmen, age thirty-nine, had a history of yo-yo dieting and demanded scientifically substantiated facts to help her make good bone-strengthening choices.

We've found that much of the anxiety and distress about osteopenia results from a lack of knowledge about this disease. Not only are there fears about what years of detrimental dieting might have done to diminish bone strength, but the uncertainty of which foods will increase or decrease bone density can be overwhelming. While a quick dietary fix to reduce your risk of fracture may not be possible, you can make easy adjustments to your daily dietary choices, which will benefit your bones over a period of time. We'll show you how.

No matter what your history with weight problems or food, this third step in the *Bone-Building Program* will give you the incentive you need to make simple bone-strengthening choices that can prevent osteopenia and fractures. Research on diet's effects on boosting bone density has confirmed that even women diagnosed with osteopenia after a fracture can improve the strength of their bones by eating certain foods.

Getting Started

In our practice, we have found that women who are hesitant to take medications to prevent osteopenia are quite willing to alter their diets with natural foods in order to prevent bone loss and fractures. So, let's get started!

Depending on your risk factors for osteopenia (review the list on page 15), you may need to make only a few adjustments to what you normally eat. Maybe you currently get adequate calcium in your diet but might benefit from soy foods high in phytoestrogens, the naturally occurring plant compounds that have some similarities to estradiol, the most potent naturally occurring estrogen. Maybe you need to add vitamin D–fortified milk to your diet to ensure adequate stores of this bone-boosting nutrient. Perhaps increasing your servings of bone-strengthening vegetables (see page 60) such as kale, broccoli, or Swiss chard will result in increased bone strength. But if you have a lengthy history of low-calorie dieting, binge eating and purging, or have avoided dairy products most of your adult life, you might need to overhaul your eating plan completely in order to boost bone strength and prevent fractures.

What does all this mean for you? No matter what your health or dieting history, you can halt and even reverse osteopenia by making the following easy bone-strengthening choices.

Choose Bone-Building Vitamins and Minerals

In the midst of searching for a "cure" for osteopenia, there is a host of evidence that eating the right nutrients is an important bone-strengthening measure—and will make a measurable difference over your lifetime. In general, nutrients are special compounds that support the body's repair, growth, and wellness. They include vitamins, minerals, amino acids, essential fatty acids, water, and the calorie sources of carbohydrate, protein, and fat. For your Bone-Building Diet, we're going to focus on specific nutrients that are known to build bone.

But before you can take advantage of healing nutrients to help boost bone strength, you must first make two minor changes in your attitude about using food to keep bones strong:

1. *Change the way you fuel your skeleton.* We want you to think of your body's skeleton as a new car. Just as a car needs the proper fuel to make it run, your skeleton needs the exact balance of essential nutrients—vitamins, minerals, antioxidants, phytochemicals, and known and little-known nutrients—to support your body and allow you to be active. Each vitamin or mineral is crucial for keeping your skeleton functioning normally. For instance, 99 percent of the calcium in our body is in our bones. Yet the only way the body can keep its calcium stores adequate is if we constantly replenish it through food or supplementation. Without enough calcium, the body draws on calcium stores in your bones, which become thinner and more fragile. Likewise, vitamin D allows calcium to leave the

intestine and enter the bloodstream. This crucial bone-strengthening vitamin also works in the kidneys to help reabsorb calcium that otherwise would be excreted.

2. *Change dietary habits left over from youth.* If you are in your 20s, 30s, or even 40s, you probably aren't thinking about the consequences of painful and debilitating fractures. Yet preventing bone loss becomes important as medical science extends our life span—and we all want to be healthy and active for as long as we live. Persuasive research supports the fact that dietary habits in teenage years and young adulthood play a crucial role in who is at risk for osteopenia and early fractures. A steady diet consisting mainly of highly processed junk foods with empty calories instead of healthful choices just may be the trigger for early fractures.

Choose Foods with These Bone-Building Vitamins and Minerals

Vitamin C	Boron	Phosphorus
Vitamin D	Calcium	Potassium
Vitamin K	Magnesium	

Calcium

Experts have identified several key nutrients believed to play a role in the attainment of bone, including protein, vitamins C, D, and K, calcium, and phosphorus. Of all these nutrients, women today are most deficient in calcium, which is associated with low bone mass, rapid bone loss, and high fracture rates. Despite volumes of scientific studies on the need for calcium to prevent bone loss, a new American Dietetic Association (ADA) study shows that 64 percent of women don't know how much calcium they need each day. National nutrition surveys show that many women and young girls consume *less than half the amount of calcium* recommended to maintain healthy bones.

Get the amount of calcium needed for your age. In our clinics, we recommend that women age twenty-five to menopause get a total of 1,200 milligrams (mg) of calcium daily. After menopause, women should consume a total of 1,500 mg of calcium each day. (See the chart on page 62 for the exact amount of calcium per age.)

Calcium needs increase during pregnancy and breast-feeding as women need to provide enough calcium for both themselves and their babies. Most of this need for calcium occurs during the last two to three months of pregnancy with calcification of the fetal skeleton. It is thought that calcium is transferred from the mother's bones to the fetus, so it's essential that moms replenish their own calcium stores. Breast-feeding moms provide calcium for their babies' growing teeth and bones—one more reason to meet the recommended daily intake.

For pregnant and lactating women the recommendation is 1,500 mg calcium per day in three divided doses (500 mg each). The vitamin D recommendation stays the same at 400 IU (International Units) daily.

No matter what the age or life stage, most women can get the recommended amounts of calcium by having four servings of calcium-rich foods each day, including:

- Yogurt made with low-fat milk or whole milk
- A selected serving of tofu, cheese, or milk
- A selected serving of fish or broccoli
- Calcium-fortified juices, breads, and cereals
- Calcium-fortified dairy products

Low-fat milk, cheese, and yogurt are good sources of calcium and have an added benefit in that they contain lactose (a sugar found in milk) that enhances calcium absorption. Other sources of calcium include salmon with bones, sardines, and green leafy vegetables (see list on pages 61–62).

Calcium-fortified drinks and foods are good bone-building choices. You can easily choose calcium-fortified products that fit in your daily dietary plan and that will help to keep bones strong. Fortified foods have vitamins and minerals added to them. Calcium is added to foods including breakfast or power bars, cereals, yogurt, and juices.

Ounce for ounce, calcium-fortified juices provide about the same amount of calcium as milk, and in a form that is well absorbed by the body. Studies have found that drinking juices fortified with calcium may be an even better way to get calcium than drinking milk. One revealing study, reported in the June 1996 issue of the *Journal of the American College of Nutrition*, concluded that while people could absorb only about 25 to 30 percent of the calcium from drinking milk, they could absorb about 36 percent of the calcium in fortified orange juice and 42 percent in calcium-enriched apple juice.

Dieters can boost dietary calcium with healthy choices. If you are dieting and have ignored your calcium needs, a host of low-calorie foods are high in calcium. Here are a few examples:

- 1 cup low-fat, calcium-fortified milk has 500 mg calcium and 80 calories
- 1 cup nonfat yogurt has 450 mg calcium and 80 calories
- 1 cup 1 percent milk-fat yogurt has 450 mg calcium and 90 calories
- 1 cup low-fat milk has 300 mg calcium and 80 calories
- 1 cup fortified soy milk (set with calcium sulfate) has 300 mg calcium and 80 calories
- 1 cup fortified orange juice has 300 mg calcium and 109 calories
- 1 cup low-fat (1 percent) chocolate milk has 300 mg calcium and 110 calories
- 1 cup cooked white beans has 270 mg calcium and 250 calories
- 1 slice low-fat (2 percent) cheese has 250 mg calcium and 55 calories
- ½ cup tofu (set with calcium sulfate) has 200–400 mg calcium and 90–100 calories
- 1 cup kale greens (steamed) has 205 mg calcium and 30–40 calories
- 1 cup mustard greens (steamed) has 200 mg calcium and 30–40 calories
- 1 cup soybeans (cooked) has 175 mg calcium and 300 calories
- 1 cup broccoli (steamed) has 145 mg calcium and 50 calories

New findings conclude that adding calcium-rich dairy foods in a calorie-controlled diet may promote weight loss. This may give new impetus for drinking more low-fat milk each day—stronger bones and weight reduction!

Some foods can block calcium's absorption. It appears that the body's ability to absorb the calcium in foods is related to other substances that are present besides the calcium. Researchers have found that the type and amounts of sugar, and also the acid content of the drink, affect how calcium is absorbed by the body.

Other factors can interfere with calcium absorption, so it's important to be aware of these. For instance, it is thought that high amounts of fat and protein in the diet might interfere with calcium absorption. Eating an excessive amount of food that contains phosphorus and phosphates (especially common in soft drinks and many convenience foods) can result in more loss of calcium from the body because of the way the body manages phosphorus. Moderate amounts of such foods seem to be acceptable.

Also, some foods that contain calcium, such as vegetables, also contain oxalate. Green leafy vegetables such as spinach contain oxalate, which may decrease the body's absorption of calcium. In such cases, even though the food may contain calcium, it may not be as available to the body. A few studies have found evidence that high amounts of caffeine in the diet might increase calcium loss. Caffeine is present in many drinks including coffee, colas, and other soft drinks. It would be reasonable to avoid excessive intake until scientists better understand this relationship.

Plan ahead to ensure adequate calcium. You can easily incorporate high-calcium food choices in your daily diet, if you plan ahead. Add the following foods to your daily diet and keep ingredients on hand for quick, bone-building meals:

Dairy Sources

Food	Serving Size	Calcium (mg)
Milk, skim	8 oz.	302
Yogurt, low-fat fruit	8 oz.	350
Yogurt, plain	8 oz.	450
Yogurt, frozen	8 oz.	278
Cheese, American	1 oz.	202
Cheese, low-fat cottage	4 oz./½ cup	69
Cheese, cream	1 oz.	30
Cheese, cheddar	1 oz.	204
Cheese, mozzarella	1 oz.	203
Cheese, Swiss	1 oz.	273
Cheese, Parmesan	¼ cup	250
Cheese, Colby/Monterey Jack	1 oz.	200
Ice cream, low-fat	4 oz./½ cup	100
Pudding	4 oz./½ cup	150

Non-Dairy Sources and Others

Food	Serving Size	Calcium (mg)
Broccoli, cooked	4 oz./½ cup	47
Spinach, cooked	4 oz./½ cup	122
Greens, cooked	4 oz./½ cup	55
Tofu, raw, firm	4 oz./½ cup	258
Instant oatmeal	1 package	150
Pancakes, buttermilk	1	80
Sardines	2	90

Non-Dairy Sources and Others (*continued*)

Food	Serving Size	Calcium (mg)
Salmon, canned, with bones	3 oz.	203
Taco with cheese	1 large	340
Quiche with cheese	⅛ of 8-inch pie	115
Macaroni and cheese, box	1 cup	100
Pizza with cheese	⅛ of 12-inch pizza	115
Breads and cereals	1 slice or ½ cup	30
Tortilla, corn	1 medium	45
Tomato soup, with milk	8 oz.	186

While food is the best way to ensure calcium absorption in the body, if your diet is inadequate, review the information on using calcium supplements (page 98). Can you take too much calcium? Excessive amounts of calcium taken in are usually excreted by the body, but constant excess could raise the risk for some persons with kidney stones or other medical problems.

Easy Calcium Booster

Add nonfat powdered dry milk to recipes to boost the calcium content. This convenient and inexpensive product can be added to casseroles, gravy, smoothies, puddings, breads, muffins, or soups. A single tablespoon of nonfat powdered dry milk adds 52 milligrams of calcium. You can add 2 to 4 tablespoons to most recipes without altering the taste.

Recommended Calcium Intakes

Children and Young Adults	Amount mg/day
6–10 years	800–1,200
11–24 years	1,200–1,500

Adult Women	Amount mg/day
Age 25 to menopause	1,200
After menopause	1,500
Pregnant or lactating	1,200–1,500

Adult Men	Amount mg/day
Age 25–65	1,000
65 and older	1,500

Non-Dairy Foods and Calcium Equivalents

If you are a vegetarian or vegan, you can still get ample calcium in your diet. The following non-dairy foods contain enough calcium to equal an 8-oz. cup of milk:

5.7 oz. dry-roasted almonds
4 cups cauliflower
2.5 cups broccoli or white beans
2 cups rutabaga
1 cup Chinese cabbage or turnip greens
½ cup calcium-fortified tofu

Vitamin C

Vitamin C, an antioxidant, helps your body synthesize collagen—a connective substance in the body—and aids in wound healing. Although vitamin C is not thought of as a key nutrient in preventing bone loss, many epidemiological studies report a positive association between vitamin C intake and bone density.

The RDA of vitamin C for women is 75 mg daily. It is advised not to take more than 2,000 mg/day because of the risk of gastrointestinal problems. Food choices with vitamin C include citrus juices and fruits, berries, tomatoes, potatoes, green and red peppers, broccoli, and spinach.

How Much Sun Is Enough to Make Vitamin D?

People age 22 to 30 make more vitamin D than people aged 62 to 80 after being exposed to the same amount of sunlight. Check out the amount of sun necessary to make vitamin D.

State	Month	Amount of Time
Massachusetts	June	5–10 minutes midday
Florida	June	2–3 minutes

Vitamin D

Calcium relies on "boosters" to be absorbed efficiently in the body. One such booster is vitamin D, or calciferol, a fat-soluble vitamin. Vitamin D is found in food and is made in the body after exposure to ultraviolet rays from the sun.

Vitamin D has similar actions to a hormone in the body since it helps activate calcium and phosphorus, two minerals necessary for strong bones and important in keeping muscles and nerves healthy. When the body has an insufficient supply of vitamin D, the blood levels of calcium and phosphorus drop as well. Where does the body turn to get more of these much-needed minerals? You guessed it—your bones.

Loss of the minerals calcium and phosphorus is directly related to bone loss. Inadequate vitamin D is associated with decreased muscle strength and increased body sway, factors that can increase the likelihood of falls. (Up to 95 percent of hip fractures can be attributed to falls.)

Vitamin D is obtained in two ways: through the skin and from the diet. The sun's ultraviolet rays trigger vitamin D synthesis in the skin. There are studies showing that simply taking a 15 to 20-minute walk several times a week will keep most women well supplied with enough vitamin D to keep bones healthy. Because vitamin D is fat soluble, it can be stored in the body. This means that casual exposure to sunlight in the summer months might allow your body to have ample amounts of this vitamin in the winter. However, if you work in an office year-round, and your exposure to sunlight through office windows is your primary exposure, you may develop a vitamin D deficiency. Also, some studies show that using a sunscreen rated over SPF 8 reduces your ability to make vitamin D by more than 90 percent.

Although younger adults get enough sunlight throughout the day to keep this vitamin in check, new research is finding that many older adults have a problem. In comprehensive studies at the New England Medical Center that shed light on aging and bone loss, researchers found that aging reduces the capacity of the skin to use sunlight to produce vitamin D.

Other factors that might cause a vitamin D deficiency include:

- Limited exposure to ultraviolet light from working indoors, using sunscreens, living in northern latitudes, or in smoggy areas
- Increased age. The gastrointestinal tract is less able to absorb vitamin D, and aging skin becomes less efficient at converting vitamin D to calcitriol, the hormone that stimulates the intestinal absorption of calcium
- Certain medications, such as anticonvulsants, can increase the breakdown and excretion of vitamin D

- Disorders associated with fat malabsorption (e.g., Crohn's disease) because vitamin D is fat soluble
- Kidney and liver diseases, which impair the ability of these organs to convert vitamin D to calcitriol

The daily intake of vitamin D should be 400 IU. Some experts suggest that those over age fifty take 400 IU of vitamin D year-round to ensure they get enough of this crucial bone-building nutrient. Daily vitamin D supplements of 400 to 800 IU per day for those sixty-five and older are also suggested. Before you go out and stock up on supplemental vitamin D, talk to your doctor first about your specific vitamin needs. If taken in excess, vitamin D might be toxic, causing symptoms of vomiting, kidney stones, and muscle weakness.

Choose Foods High in Vitamin D

Food labels list the vitamin D content as a "%DV." The DV, or Daily Value, is 400 International Units (IU). So a food with 20 percent of the DV for vitamin D contains about 80 IU.

Food Sources	Vitamin D (IU)
Halibut (3 oz.)	680
Pink salmon (canned, ¼ cup)	400
Tuna (canned, ¼ cup)	130
Milk (1 cup)	100
Minute Maid Calcium +Vit. D Orange Juice (8 oz.)	10
Yoplait Light Yogurt (6 oz.)	80
Parkay Calcium Plus (1 Tbs.)	60
Breakfast cereal, fortified (1 cup average)	40

Vitamin K
Vitamin K is an essential vitamin that may play a vital role in calcium absorption and an indirect role in preventing low bone density. The Framingham Osteoporosis Study, a cohort that was part of the Framingham Heart Study in Framingham, Massachusetts, took bone density measurements at the hip and spine in 1,112 men and 1,479 women. Using the results, researchers concluded that low dietary vitamin K intake was associated with low bone mineral density in women. This finding is consistent

with previous reports that low dietary vitamin K intake is associated with an increased risk of hip fracture.

The Nurses' Health Study, a study of 120,000 registered nurses that began in 1976 with funding from the National Institutes of Health, reported in the January 1999 *American Journal of Clinical Nutrition* that women who get at least 110 micrograms of vitamin K daily are 30 percent less likely to fracture a hip than women who ingest less than 110 micrograms. From the results of this study, researchers concluded that simply eating a serving of lettuce or other green leafy vegetable once a day might cut the risk of hip fracture in half when compared with eating one serving a week.

The RDA for vitamin K is 65 to 80 micrograms, and the best food sources include green leafy vegetables, soybean oil, broccoli, alfalfa, cooked spinach, and fish oil.

Vitamin A—How Much Is Too Much?

While vitamin A is crucial for healthy bones, some studies conclude that too much vitamin A is linked to bone loss and the risk of hip fracture. In the January 2, 2002, issue of the *Journal of the American Medical Association,* researchers reported that excessive vitamin A, particularly from retinol, may contribute to the development of osteoporotic hip fractures in women. It is also thought that too much vitamin A may interfere with vitamin D, which plays an important role in preserving bone.

Retinol is one of the most active, or usable, forms of vitamin A, and is found in animal foods such as liver and eggs and in some fortified food products. The RDA of vitamin A (retinol) for women is 2,330 International Units or IU (2,565 IU for pregnant women and 4,335 IU for lactating women). It is advisable not to take over 10,000 International Units of vitamin A (retinol) daily.

Choose Trace Minerals Necessary for Bone Strength

If you are eating a well-balanced, nutritious diet, there is probably no need to worry about a mineral deficiency. Still, it may be helpful for you to understand the function of trace minerals on bone mass and to identify the specific foods that contain these. Although the specific role trace elements play in bone loss has not been defined, they are essential for normal growth and development of bones and play a prominent role in bone metabolism and bone turnover. Let's look at a few key bone-strengthening minerals.

Phosphorus

Not only is phosphorus a key mineral in almost all chemical reactions in the body, it also works side by side with calcium to build strong bones and teeth. In fact, almost 85 percent of phosphorus is in the bone. Scientists know that as calcium increases in the body, phosphorus decreases. For most women this is not a problem. Yet, if your diet is already low in phosphorus and high in calcium, the calcium supplementation may aggravate a phosphorus deficiency, resulting in bone loss.

The RDA for phosphorus is 800 mg for adults (1,200 mg for pregnant and lactating women). It is estimated that about 10 percent of women age 60 to 80 and 15 percent of women over age 80 get less than 70 percent of the recommended daily intake of phosphorus. You can find phosphorus in fish, poultry, meats, grains, eggs, seeds, and nuts. An extra serving of milk each day can ensure that your calcium and phosphorus levels stay balanced.

Potassium

Studies show that potassium reduces calcium loss and may help prevent bone loss and fractures. In the May 2002 issue of the *Journal of Endocrinology and Metabolism*, researchers reported that the impact on bone health of a diet high in salt could be potentially harmful because salt increases urinary calcium loss. The study, performed on postmenopausal women, concluded that the consumption of excessive salt increased the level of bone minerals excreted through urine. We believe this study is of particular concern because most Americans eat more than twice as much sodium chloride as recommended by the National Institutes of Health.

Although there is no recommended daily allowance (RDA) for potassium, it is thought that consuming 2 to 2.5 grams of potassium a day is adequate. The alkaline salts in potassium occur naturally in fruits and vegetables and intervene when sodium is consumed. Therefore, a diet high in potassium-rich foods could possibly reduce calcium excretion. Foods high in potassium include bananas, orange and grapefruit juice, tomatoes, sweet potatoes, broccoli, kale, figs, raisins, chickpeas and butter beans, peanut butter, and wheat products.

Magnesium

Magnesium is involved in a number of activities supporting bone strength, preservation, and remodeling. Findings indicate that magnesium deficiency may be a risk factor for postmenopausal osteoporosis. This may be because magnesium deficiency alters calcium metabolism and the hormone that regulates calcium.

Most people get ample magnesium from their daily diet. The recommended dosages of magnesium range from 280 mg for women and 350 mg for men. Food sources include cereals, nuts, sunflower seeds, tofu, and dairy products, bananas, pineapples, plantains, raisins, artichokes, avocados, lima beans, spinach, okra, beet greens, oysters, halibut, mackerel, grouper, cod, and sole.

Boron

Boron, another mineral plentiful in fruits and vegetables, appears to play an active role in the metabolism of calcium and bone development. Although still controversial, research by the U.S. Department of Agriculture indicates that boron increases estrogen levels in the blood. As such, some researchers believe that this mineral might enhance estrogen's effects in women who take estrogen replacement therapy, and it may be helpful in retaining calcium and magnesium.

Although there is no established recommendation for boron, you can get this mineral in plentiful amounts through vegetables (particularly parsley), legumes (dried beans and peas), dried fruits, seeds, and nuts. Avoid taking megadoses with supplements since there can be side effects such as headache.

Other Trace Minerals Important for Bone Strength

- *Fluoride*—a bone-strengthening mineral that accumulates in new bone formation sites, resulting in a net gain in bone mass. Food sources of fluoride include anchovies (with bones), fluoridated drinking water, milk, salmon (with bones), sardines (with bones), tea, and vegetables grown in soil high in fluoride. (Fluoride is not to be taken in excessive amounts.)
- *Manganese*—a bone-strengthening mineral and antioxidant involved in bone and connective tissue development. Some researchers feel that this trace mineral may be as important as calcium in building bone. Food sources include eggs, green vegetables, lentils, meat, nuts, seeds, strawberries, sweet potatoes, tea, and whole grain products.
- *Zinc*—a bone-strengthening mineral crucial to building optimal bone in children. It is part of the structure of bones and is necessary

for bones to rebuild. Food sources include almonds, black-eyed peas, crab, meat, milk, peanut butter, seafood, sunflower seeds, tofu, and wheat germ.

Choose Bone-Strengthening Phytoestrogens

Phytoestrogens (PEs) are natural compounds that include isoflavones, lignans, and coumestans. These plant ingredients are present in many foods, including beans, sprouts, cabbage, spinach, soybeans, and grains, and mimic the hormone estrogen, yet appear to have no harmful side effects and may even provide a bonus in helping to prevent bone loss.

For years, soybeans have played an integral part in Asian cultures, with much lower occurrences of heart disease, breast cancer, prostate cancer, and osteoporosis rates for Asian men and women than for Americans. In Asia, consumption of legumes such as soybeans and lentils provides 25 to 45 mg of total isoflavones a day. In Japan, soy consumption is particularly high—up to 200 mg daily of isoflavones are consumed. (In Western countries, less than 5 mg a day of isoflavones are consumed.) With a diet high in soy and isoflavones, Japanese women have blood levels of phytoestrogens ten to forty times higher than those of their Western peers. In fact, breast cancer (and prostate cancer) rates for the Japanese are four times lower than for those in the United States.

While the studies are few, findings support that eating soy foods strengthens bone. For example, in a study on Chinese women who were just a few years postmenopausal, published in October 2003 in the journal *Osteoporosis International*, researchers concluded that soybean and isoflavone ingestion results in a modest but significant increase in hip bone mineral density and higher overall body bone mineral density. Asian women have a lower rate of bone loss and fractures than Western women, even though Asian women's bones are much thinner and their calcium intake is lower than that of Westerners.

Three Classes of Dietary Phytoestrogens
The three main classes of dietary phytoestrogens are isoflavones, lignans, and coumestans:

- **Isoflavones** (genistein, daidzein, glycitein, and equol) are primarily found in soybeans and soy products, chickpeas, and other legumes.

- **Lignans** (enterolactone and enterodiol) are found in oilseeds (primarily flaxseed), cereal bran, legumes, and alcohol (beer and bourbon).
- **Coumestans** (coumestrol) can be found in alfalfa and clover.

Soybean protein, soy isoflavones, genistein, daidzein, and coumestrol have all been found to have a protective effect on bone in animals that had surgical removal of the ovaries. Although the human studies are conflicting, most experts recommend eating soy foods for the isoflavone bone-boosting benefit.

Calling All Vegetarians and Vegans

If you follow a vegetarian or vegan diet or if you are lactose intolerant, it's often hard to be sure you get ample calcium and other bone-strengthening nutrients. Researchers have found that the calcium in soy milk is not as easily used by the body as the calcium in cows' milk. In fact, they conclude that it takes about 500 mg of calcium in the fortified soy milk to equal 300 mg of calcium in cows' milk. (Unfortified soy milk contains only about 10 mg of calcium per serving.) If you rely on soy milk as your primary source of calcium, drink about twice as much as you would of cows' milk to get adequate calcium.

Select from the following non-dairy sources of calcium: calcium-fortified soy or rice beverages, calcium-set tofu, calcium-fortified fruit juices, broccoli, bok choy, almonds, and calcium-fortified breakfast cereals and protein bars.

Choose Whole Foods

Although isoflavone supplements are available over the counter, there are no human studies on the long-term effects of taking large doses of purified isoflavones. That's why we recommend eating whole soy foods such as tofu, soy milk, and edamame (a green vegetable soybean), which are good sources of fiber, B vitamins, calcium, and omega-3 essential fatty acids, all important food components. Soybeans contain about 2 to 4 mg of isoflavone per gram of protein. Soy milk and tofu contain about 2 mg of isoflavone per gram of protein.

Soy protein is also available in a variety of tasty prepared foods. Check in your grocer's freezer for soy "fake" corn dogs, chicken, hamburger patties, sausage, and bacon, among others.

Calculating the Isoflavones in Soy Products

Type of Food	Isoflavones in Milligrams
Boiled soybeans	54
Tofu	28
Soy hot dogs	15
Soy milk	10
Soy mozzarella cheese	8
Soy sausage	4

Source: U.S. Department of Agriculture

The following soy products represent just a few that are available at most supermarkets:

- Isolated soy protein—a powdered soy protein that can be added to other foods such as casseroles, pasta dishes, drinks, and more. One ounce contains approximately 23 grams of soy protein.
- Soya flour—a finely ground powder that is milder in taste than soy flour. One-half cup provides 20 grams of soy protein.
- Soybeans—dried soybeans that have a nutty flavor and can be used in recipes such as baked beans or chili. Soak the beans before cooking (like any dried bean). You can add to soups or use in any recipe that calls for lentils. One-half cup provides 14.3 grams of soy protein.
- Soy flour—a very fine powder made from ground roasted soybeans. You can purchase soy flour in defatted, low-fat, natural, or full-fat versions. One-half cup of full-fat soy flour contains 15 grams of soy protein, and defatted soy flour has 24 grams of soy protein. Use soy flour to replace up to one-quarter of regular flour in recipes.
- Soy granules—nutty-textured granules that shake directly out of the container. You can soak these, then use for filler in recipes or sprinkle directly on food, such as ice cream or yogurt. Soy granules have 23 grams of soy protein per one-quarter cup.
- Soy milk—a liquid that can be used as a substitute for milk in virtually any recipe. Soy milk contains 10 grams of soy protein per 8-ounce glass. Be sure to look for soy milk that is calcium fortified.
- Tempeh—a thin cake made from fermented soybeans. Tempeh has an interesting nutty or smoky taste and chewy texture. Four ounces of tempeh contain almost 17 grams of soy protein. Tempeh is frequently used as a substitute for beef and contains more whole soybeans and fiber than soy milk or tofu.

- Textured soy protein (TVP)—a frozen, quick-cooking meat substitute made from low-fat soy flour. TVP is used as a beef substitute for burgers, chili, sloppy Joes, and more. It is available in many forms, including strips, chunks, flakes, and granules. One-half cup serving has 11 grams of soy protein. (Veggie burgers made with soy protein may or may not have isoflavones since some processed soy foods have had the isoflavones removed.)
- Tofu—a popular soy product, also called bean curd. Tofu is a tasteless food, but by blending it with herbs, spices, and other foods, it becomes very appetizing. It comes in a myriad of varieties, including soft, firm, extra firm, and silken, and it is available in regular and low-fat forms, too. Four ounces of firm tofu contain 9 to 13 grams of soy protein; the same amount of soft tofu contains 9 grams of soy protein.

Foods High in Isoflavones

Food	Serving	Isoflavones (mg)	Calories	Fat (g)
Nutlettes*	½ cup	122	140	1.5
Roasted soy nuts	¼ cup	62	195	9.5
Tempeh	½ cup	35	165	6.0
Low-fat tofu	½ cup	35	45–75	1.5–2.5
Regular tofu	½ cup	35	105–120	5.5–6.5
Soy milk	1 cup	30	120–150	4.0
Low-fat soy milk	1 cup	20	90–120	2.0

*Nutlettes is a crunchy breakfast cereal that can be ordered from Dixie USA, Inc., at (800) 347–3494. It provides 25 grams of soy protein per ½ cup.

Choose Foods High in Flavonoids

Flavonoids are the four thousand compounds responsible for the colors of fruits and flowers. These disease-fighting antioxidants have a healing effect in the body. A few studies show that the intake of flavonoids is directly linked to stronger bones. For example, there is good evidence that sipping tea instead of other drinks may help to ward off painful fractures. In a study published in 2001 in the journal *Drugs under Experimental and Clinical Research*, researchers identified resveratrol and trans-resveratrol, two powerful phytoestrogens present in the skins of grapes and other plant foods and wine, as demonstrating a broad spectrum of pharmacological health benefits. These phytoestrogens may be a possible alternative to hormone replacement therapy (HRT) for bone formation and osteoporosis prevention.

In another revealing study, published in May 2002 in the journal *Archives of Internal Medicine*, scientists found that men and women who drank tea for years had denser bones at three different skeletal sites, regardless of the type or amount of tea they consumed each day. Researchers concluded that drinking tea regularly for at least ten years was estimated to boost bone mineral density by up to 5 percent. This bone-boosting benefit may be attributed to special compounds in tea—such as fluoride, phyto-estrogens, and flavonoids, a group of antioxidants—all working together. Some key prevention benefits of tea include the following:

- Antioxidant
- Antibacterial
- Antivirus
- Anti-aging properties
- Anti-inflammatory

Just Say No to Cola

Some new findings presented at the 25th Annual Meeting of the American Society for Bone and Mineral Research in September 2003 concluded that colas, but not other carbonated soft drinks, contribute to the loss of bone mineral density in adult women. Researchers thought this was because of calcium-binding phosphoric acid in colas and because sometimes carbonated soft drinks displace milk or calcium-fortified juices in the diet. While phosphoric acid is present in other food sources, including dairy products, it's thought that it does not cause the same sort of problem.

In the study, 1,672 women and 1,148 men were evaluated over a period of five years, from 1996 to 2001. The group was divided into two groups, those who consumed cola daily and those who drank cola (or other sorts of carbonated beverages including clear sodas) once a week or less. BMD measurements were taken at the spine and three sites of the hip. Among the female subjects, regular cola drinkers had decreased BMD compared with the infrequent drinkers.

Researchers concluded that drinking more than one 12-ounce cola daily resulted in significantly lower bone mineral density in the hip. It is thought that with cola drinks, you get the extra doses of phosphoric acid without any calcium. This extra phosphorus binds with calcium and prevents it from being absorbed in the body.

Four Weeks to Better Bones

Plan to incorporate the following bone-strengthening food suggestions in your daily meal plan over the next four weeks. By trying just one new food or bone-strengthening recipe (see page 148 to 186) each day, you can easily get accustomed to adding these key nutrients in your regular diet.

Week 1: Bone-Strengthening Suggestions

Monday	Try the Grilled Salmon with Fresh Herbs (page 166) for a calcium boost tonight.
Tuesday	Creamy Artichoke Dip (page 179) is filled with bone-building nutrients. Make this dip and enjoy with raw vegetables or crackers.
Wednesday	Make a bone-strengthening smoothie for breakfast by combining 6 ounces calcium-fortified orange juice, 4 ounces soy milk, ½ banana, and ½ cup fresh or frozen strawberries. Add honey to taste.
Thursday	Buy cottage cheese that is calcium-fortified and then add chopped vegetables such as red and green bell peppers, carrots, and green onions for a delicious, bone-building lunch.
Friday	Try a calcium-fortified yogurt for a snack today. Yogurt has more calcium per ounce than milk and is a good source of protein and other nutrients.
Saturday	Add 1 slice of provolone or smoked cheese to your Saturday morning omelet. Drink calcium-fortified orange juice for an extra boost to your bone health.
Sunday	Try two new bone-building and kid-pleasing recipes today. Peanut Butter and Jelly Shake, page 150, and Strawberry Muffins, page 150, are well loved by young and old!

Week 2: Bone-Strengthening Suggestions

Monday	Mother Mac's Elegant Carrots, page 176, is a delicious recipe that is a meal in itself. Loaded with bone-building cheese, you can complement the dish with fresh bread and a green leafy salad. Top your salad with chickpeas for added protein and bone-building nutrients.

Tuesday	Make Mom's Baked Beans, page 183, and substitute your favorite beans in this dish. Chickpeas, butter beans, lentils, and other beans are high in bone-building nutrients.
Wednesday	Serve salmon for dinner and top with ½ cup white beans. Add ½ cup steamed broccoli topped with 1 slice low-fat cheese.
Thursday	Add ½ cup cooked edamame (green soybeans found in your grocer's freezer) to your lunch or dinner salad. They make a tasty addition and give a bone-strengthening boost. Top the salad with fresh mozzarella cheese.
Friday	Have an evening snack of low-fat sharp cheddar cheese slices wrapped around apple strips.
Saturday	Sprinkle baked tortilla chips with shredded cheese. Heat in microwave oven until cheese melts. Add chopped lettuce, tomatoes, green onions, and black olives for a fun, bone-strengthening snack.
Sunday	Summer Squash Gratin, page 178, is the perfect accompaniment to any meal. The added cheese makes this healthy dish a bone-building superstar.

Week 3: Bone-Strengthening Suggestions

Monday	Eat an all-vegetable dinner tonight. Include several of the vegetables that are loaded with calcium such as broccoli, Brussels sprouts, mustard greens, kale, or Swiss chard.
Tuesday	Serve the Creamy Tomato Soup, page 156, tonight for dinner. Add a fresh green salad and grate Parmesan cheese on top for an added bone boost.
Wednesday	Fettucine Alfredo, page 163, is a delicious side dish or bone-building main dish for vegetarians.
Thursday	Try Gardenburger, Boca Burger, or Morningstar Farm brands soy products available in your grocer's freezer. These soy products are "meat-mimics" and can be used in place of chicken, sausage, bacon, or ground beef. Read the label to see how much calcium is provided per serving.
Friday	Seafood Chowder, page 153, is high in bone-building calcium and satisfying when eaten with wheat crackers and a fresh green salad.

Saturday	Add low-fat grated cheese to your lunch or dinner salad. Grate cheese on top of soups or add a slice of low-fat Swiss cheese to your ham sandwich.
Sunday	Baked Spaghetti, page 172, is an all-time favorite for most families. This is an easy way to please your kids' tastes and help to strengthen their bones, too.

Week 4: Bone-Strengthening Suggestions

Monday	Add powdered skim milk to your daily smoothie today and see how easy it is to up your calcium count without adding to your daily caloric intake.
Tuesday	Fresh greens are high in calcium and a healthy addition to the diet. Try the Penne Pasta with Stir-Fry Greens, one of our new bone-building recipes on page 162.
Wednesday	Blend 1 package silken tofu with 1 packet onion soup mix for a bone-strengthening dip. Use with fresh vegetable strips or crackers.
Thursday	Read the package label to make sure the power bar you eat is high in calcium. Be sure to drink plenty of fluids to aid in absorption of nutrients and maintain hydration.
Friday	Make a special cranberry fruit smoothie with 1 cup vanilla soy milk, ½ large banana, 2 tablespoons frozen cranberry juice concentrate (undiluted), and ¼ cup strawberries. Blend until smooth.
Saturday	Enjoy a light dessert with an extra calcium boost by making no-sugar prepared pudding with low-fat milk.
Sunday	Use bok choy raw in your lunch or dinner salad, or sauté it in a stir-fry with other bone-strengthening vegetables.

Bone-Strengthening Shopping List

Be sure to keep the following foods on hand for quick recipes:

Low-fat milk
Low-fat yogurt
Low-fat ice cream
Buttermilk
Low-fat cheese
Cottage cheese
Ricotta cheese
Evaporated skim milk (canned)
Nonfat milk powder (dry)

Edamame (green soybeans found in your grocer's freezer that can be
   used in soups, salads, rice and pasta dishes)
Calcium-fortified orange juice
Calcium-enriched bread
Calcium-fortified cereal
Macaroni and cheese (boxed or frozen)
White beans (canned or dry)
Salmon with bones
Sardines with bones

CHAPTER 4

Step 4: Take Strong Steps to Prevent Fractures

Surprisingly, you have far greater control over your bone health than you've been led to believe by the popular media—and it extends beyond exercising daily and drinking milk. To reverse osteopenia, you must understand the risk factors you can control—and the ones you can't—and then make key changes to strengthen and protect your bones.

Take twenty-eight-year-old Beth, for example. This petite young attorney came to our clinic because she was concerned about her personal risk for bone loss and fractures. Both her mother and grandmother had suffered early fractures after falling, and Beth did not want to experience the same. While Beth's bone density T score was normal for her age, it was important for her to review her risk for osteopenia and take control of any risk factors she could change. Let's look at Beth's personal risk factors:

Risk Factors Beth Cannot Change	**Risk Factors Beth Can Change**
Gender (being female)	Cigarette smoking
Race (Caucasian)	Sedentary lifestyle
Weighing less than 127 pounds	Lack of dairy products in diet
Genetics (mother and grandmother)	

After checking the risk factor list on page 15, we discussed those areas Beth could change and the risk factors she had to accept. For example, we know there is a direct relationship between tobacco use and decreased bone density—smoking cigarettes doubles the risk of bone loss. So, the first risk factor Beth can change is to stop smoking. We gave her suggestions on how to quit.

Beth can also include calcium-rich foods in her diet—even if she cannot eat dairy products. As discussed in Step 3, plenty of calcium-fortified foods, as well as vegetables and soy products, are rich in this mineral and other bone-building nutrients. Adding calcium supplements is another step Beth can take to prevent bone loss and fractures. We explained how she needed at least 1,200 mg of calcium from food and supplements to stop osteopenia.

Because Beth is naturally slim, she never felt pressed to exercise for weight loss. But she needs to exercise to strengthen her bones and maintain bone density. We reviewed the suggested weight-bearing and resistance exercises in Step 2 for Beth and urged her to start this program immediately. Not only would exercise strengthen Beth's bones, but by improving her muscle strength and flexibility, exercise also would reduce her risk for falling and breaking bones.

As we've discussed, there are risk factors for osteopenia that are beyond your control. Beth can't change her genetic inheritance (both her mother and grandmother had early bone loss with fractures, putting her at a higher risk) or race (Caucasian women are at higher risk than African-American women). But she could stop smoking cigarettes, add calcium to her diet, and exercise regularly.

For Randi, a thirty-six-year-old mother of two who had a hysterectomy a few years ago without subsequent estrogen replacement therapy, taking cortisone medications for several years to control her asthma increased her risk of early bone loss and fractures. Asthma is a common lung disease that affects around 14 million Americans. While the disease itself might not pose a threat to bone health, cortisone medications (corticosteroids), used to treat the disease, in tablet form or inhaler, can have a negative impact on the bones.

Corticosteroids are anti-inflammatory medications. Although these drugs reduce inflammation, they also decrease calcium absorbed from food, increase calcium loss from the kidneys, and decrease bone formation. Corticosteroids also hinder the manufacturing of sex hormones in women and men, which contributes to bone loss. The medication in high doses can even cause muscle weakness, increasing the risk of falling.

Because Randi was aware of this drug side effect, she counteracted the bone-robbing effect of this lifesaving medication by also taking one of the bone-building medications that help to prevent bone loss and fracture (listed on page 111). Randi also made an effort to exercise daily, included more bone-building foods in her daily diet, and took extra calcium supplements as an added protection.

Another patient, thirty-three-year-old Caroline, was diagnosed with Crohn's disease, an inflammatory bowel disease (IBD), in her early twenties. About 30 to 60 percent of people with IBD may have low bone density, putting them at significant risk for fractures. (Other diseases, such as hyperthyroidism, alcoholism, chronic kidney disease, lactose intolerance, liver disease, and others, also increase the risk for fractures.)

Caroline cannot change having this illness, but she can take preventive measures for osteopenia by exercising daily, following a bone-building diet, and taking calcium supplements. If Caroline ever needs to take prednisone for more than three months, we will consider prescribing one of the safe bone-building medications, discussed in Step 5. Caroline has a bone density test every two years to assess her bone health. So far, by following these proactive strategies, she has avoided fractures.

Any Woman Can Keep Bones Strong

No matter what your risk of osteopenia, we believe that any woman can reverse osteopenia and keep bones strong. In Step 4, we want to identify four common bone robbers you can control—and change. Not only do the following bone robbers increase your risk of fractures, they can affect your total well-being:

1. Excessive alcohol consumption
2. Smoking
3. The female athlete triad (osteopenia, amenorrhea, and eating disorders)
4. Falls, which increase your risk of fracture

Let's look in detail at these bone robbers and how they influence your risk of fracture. Then, we want you to consider some bone-building strategies that will give you an added boost of confidence that you're doing all you can to reverse osteopenia and prevent painful fractures.

Excessive Alcohol Consumption

Excessive alcohol consumption is a serious risk factor for early bone loss and fractures. At our clinic, we see younger and younger women with early bone loss and fractures because of excessive alcohol consumption. If you drink more than two or three drinks daily (considered "heavy" drinking), this is also linked to an increased risk of menstrual problems and early menopause, as well as bone loss.

Many of our patients affected with early bone loss from heavy alcohol consumption report feeling pain in the back, along with fractures. This is because alcohol's deleterious effect on bone tissue possibly results in reduced bone formation. Mineral and hormonal metabolism can also be impaired with alcohol consumption.

Often, women who drink alcohol in excessive amounts substitute the drinks for meals and become malnourished. This further intensifies alcohol's toxic effect on bones, since a diet high in alcohol is low in nutrients. For women, alcohol may have an even more destructive effect than for men because the percentage of water is less in a woman's body. This means that the alcohol consumed is less diluted and can make a greater impact.

Alcohol disrupts the body's calcium balance in various ways. For instance, excessive alcohol consumption increases levels of the body's parathyroid hormone (PTH), an important endocrine regulator of calcium and phosphorus concentration. In cases of chronic alcohol misuse, the PTH levels stay elevated, creating a strain on the body's calcium reserves. Alcohol also inhibits the production of key liver enzymes that are necessary for converting the inactive type of vitamin D to the active type. When the body is deficient in vitamin D, there is reduced calcium absorption.

Hormonal deficiencies are another consequence of excessive alcohol consumption. In women, excessive exposure to alcohol can result in irregular menstrual cycles, which increase the possibility of osteopenia and fractures. Alcohol can also increase levels of cortisol, a stress hormone. This is linked to reduced bone formation and increased bone resorption.

Last, excessive alcohol consumption increases the risk of falling. Falls are to blame in 95 percent of all hip fractures, but this is one risk factor you can control.

Bone-Building Strategy: Although alcohol consumption is a key risk factor for early bone loss, it is one that you can change. Here is what we tell all our patients:

- If you drink alcohol, do so in moderation.
- If you don't drink, don't start now.

Recent studies have found that there may be an increase in bone mass after more than five years of stopping alcohol. This increase in bone is important to your strength in later years, so it is worth stopping alcohol now. Continue to follow the *Bone-Building Program* by exercising regularly, eating plenty of high-calcium and nutritious foods, taking medications and supplements (if needed), and getting ample vitamin D from sunlight or fortified foods.

Smoking

Most women know that cigarette smoking doubles your risk of heart disease, stroke, cancer, and lung disease. What most women do not know is that smoking doubles the chance of bone loss and fractures. One reason is that tobacco increases the rate of bone loss by reducing the effectiveness of the body's estrogen.

Women who smoke and are underweight are at even greater risk for early bone loss and fractures. Many smokers also have lung diseases such as emphysema or chronic bronchitis, causing a reduction of oxygen in the blood. This lower level of oxygen may affect the way the body builds and removes bone. Also, corticosteroids used to treat respiratory problems increase the risk of bone loss and fractures by decreasing the activity of cells that produce bone.

If you've tried to stop smoking to no avail, you're in great company. Nicotine, one of the key toxins in cigarette smoke, is highly addictive and has myriad pleasurable but hazardous effects on the brain that trigger the biologic urge to smoke. Once nicotine "hits" brain cell receptors it stimulates the release of neurotransmitters—the brain's chemical messengers. These messengers—acetylcholine, dopamine, serotonin, and beta-endorphin—affect how we pay attention, think, eat, deal with stress, and feel pleasure. Perhaps that is why some women reach for a cigarette whenever they need to feel alert, be productive, or cope with daily anxiety and tension. Most smokers are addicted to cigarettes both biologically and habitually (learned behavior).

Bone-Building Strategy: Smoking increases the risk of bone loss, in addition to respiratory problems and certain cancers. It's also an important risk factor that you can change—though you cannot control your gender or genetics, you can stop smoking.

Sometimes it takes a serious disease to make a person quit smoking. Is the threat of weak, thinning bones enough to motivate you? When you do make a commitment to stop, make a plan for coping with symptoms of withdrawal—there are ways to avoid the unpleasantness you've read and heard about.

Because of the nicotine in cigarettes, you may experience symptoms of withdrawal such as irritability, nervousness, and headaches for one to two weeks, especially if you have been a heavy smoker. We suggest that you talk with your doctor, especially if you want to try nicotine patches or chewing gum, which are available over the counter (no prescription needed) at most pharmacies or as prescriptions. The patches or chewing gum can help you through the difficult period of withdrawal, helping to make the physical problem less troublesome.

Be aware of the triggers that increase your desire for a cigarette. For instance, you may crave a cigarette with your morning coffee, after dinner, or while relaxing by the swimming pool. Try to change these vulnerable situations. Drink your coffee in a different mug and go to another room to break those old associations. Have gum to chew after mealtime so you don't immediately desire a cigarette. Suck on sugar-free candy while relaxing poolside to avoid the risk of lighting a cigarette. Also, keep several flavors of sugar-free gum in the car and limit as much as possible your access to cigarettes.

It is important to remember that even for those who have stopped smoking for years, the urge to smoke can always return. It is a matter of mental self-control to stay away from cigarettes. Having the emotional support of a spouse, family, and understanding friends and coworkers is very important.

Stop!

A study presented in the May 1999 issue of the *Journal of the American Medical Association* confirmed that exercise plays a key role in smoking cessation for women, particularly when combined with other techniques such as nicotine patches, Wellbutrin (a prescription antidepressant medication), and support groups. Use this opportunity to exercise more. Step 2 of the *Bone-Building Program* will help you to eliminate the bone-robbing habit of smoking.

No matter how low your risk factors are for osteopenia and fractures, it is vital to your overall health and the health of your bones to stop

> ### Alert!
>
> Be sure to speak to your doctor before taking any over-the-counter nicotine medications if you are pregnant, breast-feeding, or have serious heart trouble.

smoking. Soon after quitting, your ability to exercise will increase, which is another risk factor you can gain control over. If you have trouble stopping, talk to your doctor or call your local chapter of the American Lung Association or the American Cancer Society.

Female Athlete Triad

We talked about eating disorders at length in Step 3 and how this increasing problem among young women is contributing to early bone loss. We now know that there is a female athlete triad, which refers to three factors that may be deleterious to female athletes:

1. Osteopenia
2. Amenorrhea (loss of menstrual periods)
3. Eating disorders

Today many active women excel in sports and exercise at high levels. One of our patients, Keri, a thirty-two-year-old mother and physical therapist, runs several marathons each year. When Keri's not running, she cross-trains and participates in adventure racing, which combines trail-running, mountain biking, and kayaking/canoeing. Keri watches her diet, making sure she gets ample calcium and other bone-building nutrients, and backs off her rigorous training schedule when she begins to get too thin. Because Keri is educated about osteopenia and the female athlete triad specifically, she works to maintain a healthy balance between athletic training and keeping her bones strong and body functioning normally.

We've witnessed in our practice that the female athlete triad is increasingly common among younger women who are overly concerned with body image or being at a low body weight. Researchers have found that runners are at higher risk for fractures, especially during active training periods. Young female athletes who train intensely are at greater risk for menstrual disturbances and stress fractures. Some research identifies female track and field athletes with stress fractures as being likely to have delayed onset of menstrual periods, menstrual irregularities, and low bone density. These findings suggest that female athletes in intense training may need a higher level of bone density than other women to avoid stress fractures. A bone density test may be a good idea for female athletes who have a high level of training, especially runners and those who have had one or more stress fractures.

Most female and male athletes are concerned about their body weight and shape, and may have a strict diet to keep their weight low. Again, this is especially true for runners. Avoiding meat to keep weight down is a common practice among some athletes. In this case, researchers have pointed out that avoiding key nutrients could lead to less than adequate amounts of protein, iron, calcium, and zinc in the diet.

Bone-Building Strategy: If you are at risk for the female athlete triad, it's important to review your risk factors for osteopenia and minimize or correct what you can. Be vigilant as to how training affects your body and consult your doctor if you stop menstruating or if body fat decreases below 12 percent. Athletes with menstrual disorders have lower estrogen levels, which often leads to lower bone mass. Research findings show that a young woman who hasn't menstruated in four years may have the bone density of a fifty-year-old woman.

Increase calcium in the diet (or through supplementation), and get plenty of calories to avoid dangerously low weight or body fat levels. Anything below 12 percent for the female athlete is incompatible with strong bones. Talk to your doctor about getting a bone density test annually to assess your bone mass. Check with your gynecologist about ways to correct irregular periods. Consulting with a sports medicine specialist may also be helpful. Many times non-weight-bearing exercise, such as swimming, may be prescribed so you can maintain aerobic fitness while the fracture heals. Medications to improve bone strength may also be useful.

Avoiding Falls

While falls are not "bone robbers" per se, they can rob you of an active life if the result is a debilitating fracture. And falls are a serious concern when it comes to osteopenia.

You might think that you're too young to worry about falls and think your bones are strong enough to support the trauma without injury. That's not always true. We've treated teenage gymnasts and runners who have suffered painful fractures after a fall. One young woman suffered a fall when she slipped down the stairs in her cotton socks before a college track meet. The slip resulted in two fractures that kept her from competing the entire season. Another twenty-two-year-old patient tripped on her toddler's blocks and fell on her wrist. Again, a careless fall led to a painful fracture and weeks of rehabilitation. Because osteopenia progresses without any symptoms at all, falls are dangerous for women of any age who are unaware that they have low bone density.

Let's review the facts about falls:

- Falls are a leading cause of injury and fractures.
- More than 11 million older adults (one of three) in the United States fall each year.
- One in ten falls causes a serious injury.
- At least 95 percent of hip fractures nationwide are caused by falls. (Frighteningly, one-quarter of hip fracture patients die within a year; 40 percent need a nursing home; and half who get to rehabilitation never walk without assistance again.)

Carmen, a thirty-seven-year-old mother of two, had a history of falling. "If anyone is going to trip, it is usually me," she said. "I've tripped over our new puppy, my son's bicycle, and on a loose board on our wooden decks. I even slipped and fell down the stairs at my mother's house while trying to balance a basket of laundry and a box of books."

Now that Carmen has been diagnosed with osteopenia, she realizes that she must protect herself from these careless falls or else suffer with the consequences of painful fractures. She is following the strategies to safeguard her home and lawn. Following is her line of attack against falls.

Fall-Proof the Front Lawn and Home Entry

- Keep garden hoses coiled when not in use and tuck them next to the house. Some garden hoses automatically recoil when not in use, which can save you time and decrease your risk of tripping.
- Make sure sprinkler heads are clearly marked and visible.
- Level uneven spots in the lawn.
- Make sure the sidewalk is level leading to the front door. Fill in any cracks in the sidewalk and level uneven places.
- Keep the entrance doormat flat on the ground and make sure it has no curled or frayed edges.

- Keep all children's toys stored properly after use.
- Have proper lighting during evening hours so the walkway is clearly visible.

Fall-Proof the Living Room

- Keep the foyer or entrance of your home free of obstructions.
- Replace any frayed rugs or uneven wood or tiles.
- Check the living room lighting and make sure it is adequate. If you are forty or older, you might need two to three times as much illumination as a younger adult.
- Make sure there are no telephone cords or lamp cords in heavily trafficked areas or pathways.
- Hem any drapes or curtains that are too long and might cause a potential problem.
- Make certain that tables, chairs, and couches are the proper height (your hips should never be lower than your knees).
- Secure rugs so they cannot be lifted (adhesive carpet strips are available at any home or carpet store).
- Feel the carpet for raised spots that might throw you off balance.

Fall-Proof the Stairway and Hallway

- Make sure your stairs are well lighted.
- Have a solid banister or railing and use it.
- Always wear shoes when using the stairs to give you traction.
- Remove any clutter or throw rugs that could block the walkway of the stairs.
- Make sure your robe or pajamas aren't so long that they trip you— on the stairs or anywhere else.
- Put a small basket or plastic carrier off to the side of the stairs to put items in to carry up and down, so you can still hold on to the banister.

Fall-Proof the Bathroom

- Purchase a rubber bath mat that runs the length of the tub and has a nonslip surface.
- Make sure the floor has a nonskid surface with carpeting or a nonskid bath mat.

Fall-Proof the Kitchen

- Put cabinet or pantry shelves on casters so the items are easy to access.
- As with all rooms in your home, make sure the kitchen lighting is bright, using the highest wattage bulb your system can handle.

Fall-Proof the Bedroom

- Make sure your bedroom lighting is adequate, especially at nighttime. Have a reliable light next to your bed, and leave a closet light on at night or have a nightlight in the hallway. Put a flashlight in your nightstand in case of power outage or if you still have trouble seeing at night.
- Remove all clutter. Make sure your bedspread or comforter fits tightly and does not slip off the bed. The dust ruffle should clear the floor.
- If you have wood floors, do not use a cleaner that adds shine and creates a slippery surface.
- Never use a decorative rug next to your bed, since these rugs can easily slide when stepped on.

Fall-Proof Your Pet

- If you have a small pet, fasten bells to its collar so you will know where it is even in a dark room.

Other Fall-Proofing Tips

- *Check your medications.* Talk to your doctor or pharmacist about medication side effects. Make sure you know if your medications can have a negative interaction with alcohol. If so, avoid alcoholic beverages as these might increase the chance of falling. If you are taking more than one medication, make sure there is no negative interaction that could cause dizziness or disorientation.
- *Get annual vision checks.* Make sure your glasses or contact lenses are the correct strength.
- *Stay flexible.* Continue the Bone-Building Workout in Step 2, and consider learning tai chi or yoga to increase flexibility and balance.
- *Fall the right way, if possible.* Try to fall forward or to land on your buttocks during a fall. A hip fracture is more likely to occur if you fall to either side.

Remember, these proactive fall-proofing steps will allow you to avoid mishaps that could undo all the progress you've made with your *Bone-Building Program*. It will just take an hour or two to ensure your optimal safety—and the long-term results will be well worth it.

Medications That Can Increase the Risk of Falling

- Antidepressants
- Pain medications
- Muscle relaxers
- Anti-anxiety medications
- Blood pressure medication
- Heart medicines
- Diuretics or water pills

Wear Shoes That Fit

Your feet are the foundation upon which your body rests, so avoid ill-fitting shoes that increase your risk of fractures. If your shoes are too tight or too loose or the heels are too high, you have a greater chance of losing your footing and falling.

So, what kind of shoe is best? Depending on their situation, we recommend that patients wear a sturdy flat shoe that supports their weight yet does not cause the body to be imbalanced. When selecting running shoes, we suggest that women choose nonstick soles, a shoe with adequate shock absorption, and purchase new shoes every 350 to 400 miles, so the shoes don't wear down in key support areas. We know that shoe age—not shoe cost—is crucial in preventing stress fractures for athletes. In addition, running shoes do not have the lateral support needed for tennis, so make sure you buy the appropriate shoe for the intended sport.

CHAPTER 5

Step 5: An Integrative Medicine Approach

Following a hysterectomy with removal of her uterus and ovaries, Janie, age thirty-five, plunged into menopause—overnight. She began hormone replacement therapy with estrogen and expected to continue indefinitely. Then, in March 2004, the Women's Health Initiative study was halted because estrogen replacement had been linked to an increased stroke risk. Janie stopped the medication immediately.

This young mother had read in a women's magazine that going off estrogen "cold turkey" could result in a rapid loss of bone. Because she had been diagnosed with osteopenia already, she didn't know what to do and was frightened about the possible consequences.

Lisa, age forty-three, had a family history of early menopause and osteoporosis. Both her mother and aunt went through menopause in their mid-40s, which was followed by fractures before age fifty. At 5'2" and weighing around 100 pounds, Lisa was underweight and had a very small frame. She also smoked, which increased her chance for osteopenia. While opposed to hormone replacement therapy, Lisa feared the loss of estrogen might accelerate bone loss and lead all too quickly to fractures.

First Choose Prevention

No matter what your age or life stage, we believe that the best way to avoid osteopenia and fractures is to practice healthy prevention habits, as discussed in Steps 1 to 4:

Step 1: Be aware of your personal risk factors for osteopenia and getting a bone density test at the right time.

Step 2: Exercise regularly in the best way to build bone mass.

Step 3: Eat bone-strengthening foods with plenty of calcium, vitamin
D, phosphorus, and magnesium.

Step 4: Take proactive steps to prevent fractures by stopping smoking,
avoiding excess alcohol consumption, recognizing and treating the
female athlete triad, and fall-proofing your home.

But there are times when bone loss needs treatment that is more aggres-
sive in order to prevent fractures. In Step 5 we will explain the safest medications to reverse osteopenia and osteoporosis and prevent the first
fracture. We'll also give you some effective natural dietary supplements that
can be used to increase bone density and help to resolve some annoying
menopausal symptoms when that transition happens in your life.

Ages and Stages

When Ellen had her last period at age forty-nine, she called our office and
asked the nurse for a prescription for Fosamax, a bone-building medication that a friend was taking to prevent fractures. We reviewed Ellen's
chart and saw that her last bone density test was in a normal range for her
age with a T score of −1.0. This active mother of three teenagers walked
several miles each day, maintained a healthy weight, didn't smoke, and
was not on any medications. Actually, the only risk factor Ellen had for
osteoporosis was starting menopause. Other than that, Ellen was an energetic and strong woman.

Dr. Harris explained to Ellen that fractures don't just happen during
the month of your last menstrual period. It takes years for bone thinning
to destroy your bones. That's why the 5-Step *Bone-Building Program* is so
important for younger women—to help you build the strongest bones
possible before menopause, so you have extra "stores" when bone loss
does happen.

More than forty-two million women in America are over fifty right
now, making this the largest group of women in history to hit menopause
at the same time. We know that many of these women will live at least
one-third of their lives after menopause. Soon one person out of six will
be over age sixty-five. The number of hip and other fractures will skyrocket,

unless we all take personal responsibility and action to stay strong and healthy.

The transition from a woman's childbearing years to post-reproductive years is a natural part of life. During childbearing years, estrogen levels continue to keep bones strong for many women, but around the time that menopause begins, known as perimenopause, a process of physical change that goes on for about ten years before your last period, the ovaries' production of estrogen and progesterone becomes erratic. But when "endogenous" estrogen (the kind made by your own body) starts the dramatic decline at menopause, the bone protection is compromised and usually results in loss of bone mass.

Without estrogen, bone removal outstrips bone building and bones begin to become thinner—without any outward signs or symptoms to alert you. If the estrogen is not replaced, then after menopause your bones may continue to decrease in density until they become thin enough to break. Once you have had one fracture, you are at a much higher risk for more fractures.

Hormone Replacement Therapy

For years, younger women like Janie were given prescriptions for estrogen if they underwent a surgical hysterectomy. In fact, in 2004, more than one million American women under the age of forty were taking Premarin, the popular estrogen pill. Middle-age women like Ellen were given hormone replacement therapy (HRT), estrogen plus progesterone, by their gynecologists to slow bone loss at menopause. Doctors gave HRT as a remedy for menopausal symptoms such as hot flashes, night sweats, and vaginal dryness. HRT was also often prescribed with the expectation that it would help prevent cardiovascular disease, such as heart attack and stroke. It was almost a routine treatment for every woman at menopause.

Risks Outweigh Benefits

Then the tide changed. In 2002, researchers at the National Heart, Lung and Blood Institute (NHLBI) prematurely terminated a part of the Women's Health Initiative (WHI), a long-term study of the risks and benefits of hormone replacement therapy to reduce the occurrence of heart disease, breast and colorectal cancer, and bone fractures in healthy postmenopausal women. The study was stopped after five years because of concerns that the risks of drug therapy outweighed the benefits. While these risks were associated with combination therapy—estrogen plus progesterone, or progestin, and not with estrogen alone—the study nevertheless raised questions among some researchers about the wisdom of giving estrogen treatment alone. In 2004, the estrogen treatment portion of the study was also stopped because of the possibility of an increased risk of stroke. (Estrogen usage, with or without progesterone, approximately doubles the estrogen level of a menopausal woman. Even with HRT, the estrogen and progesterone levels may not reach the natural levels of a pre-menopausal woman.)

In the Women's Health Initiative prevention trial, more than 16,600 women aged 50 to 79 were enrolled and then randomly assigned to a daily dose of .625 mg of conjugated estrogen plus 2.5 mg of medroxy-progesterone acetate (the medications in Prempro) or to a placebo. The data that came in was not what researchers expected. The findings suggested that estrogen/progestin therapy resulted in an increased risk of heart attacks (29 percent), stroke (41 percent), venous blood clots (50 percent), and breast cancer (26 percent).

In the Women's Health Initiative Memory Study, researchers were surprised to find that estrogen plus progestin doubled the risk for developing dementia (a decline in mental ability or cognitive function) in post-menopausal women age sixty-five and older. This risk increased for all types of dementia, including Alzheimer's disease. Before this, it was often thought that HRT might actually delay or prevent Alzheimer's disease.

On a positive note, the combination HRT resulted in a decreased risk of hip fractures (34 percent) and total fractures (24 percent) and a lower risk of colon cancer (37 percent).

The Women's Health Initiative Prevention Trial
Findings on Hormone Replacement Therapy (HRT)—Risks

Increased Risk
15% increase in global index (risks exceeded benefits)
29% increase in coronary heart disease events
41% increase in stroke
111% increase in deep vein thrombosis or blood clots
22% increase in total cardiovascular disease
26% increase in invasive breast cancer

Decreased Risk
37% decrease in colorectal cancer
34% decrease in hip and clinical vertebral fractures

Estrogen Therapy Alone

Estrogen alone should not be taken unless a woman has had a hysterectomy, because estrogen alone might cause the inside lining of the uterus to become thickened and increase the risk of cancer of the uterus. While estrogen is still the most effective supplement for the common problems of hot flashes and vaginal dryness, doctors now evaluate each woman's individual risks and benefits for taking estrogen with respect to her whole health, including bone health, heart disease, stroke, and risk for certain types of cancer.

The actual numbers of increased cases of cancer, heart attack, stroke, and blood clots were relatively low in the WHI hormone study, but higher than expected. Because of this information, there must be an individual decision whether to add estrogen and progesterone or estrogen alone, based on your own symptoms and your own risks otherwise. Other medications are available to treat some of the bothersome symptoms of menopause, for example, medications such as antidepressants in the selective serotonin reuptake inhibitor class including venlafaxine (Effexor) and paroxetine (Paxil), fluoxetine (Sarafem, Prozac), blood pressure medications like clonidine (Catapres), and complementary therapies such as the herb black cohosh which may help reduce the symptoms of hot flashes, perhaps without serious side effects.

Other preparations of estrogen therapy, such as vaginal creams containing estrogen, can help with vaginal dryness, may improve bladder control, and may decrease the chance of recurrent bladder infections in some women.

Estrogen therapy can help other aspects of a woman's life by improving sleep quality due to decreased nighttime hot flashes. In some women, it may improve symptoms of depressed mood and anxiety that may come with menopause.

In the past, estrogen or estrogen plus progesterone were used to control the symptoms of menopause. Since the halt of the WHI hormone study, more than 80 percent of women have stopped their HRT because of concern of side effects.

Effective medications and treatments for the prevention and treatment of osteopenia and osteoporosis other than estrogen are available. In fact, 15 to 20 percent of women who take estrogen still lose bone. Many of the alternative treatments do not carry the same increased health risks. There are also other effective preventive measures against heart disease and stroke. In light of all that, most physicians do not routinely prescribe estrogen for prevention and treatment of osteoporosis or cardiovascular disease.

Specific Recommendations for
Use of HRT and/or Use of Estrogen Alone

For Menopausal Symptoms, Check with Your Doctor
Hormone replacement therapy, short-term (6 months to 5 years)

- estrogen or estrogen-progesterone (if you have a uterus)
- low-dose oral contraceptive if perimenopausal

Estrogen and progesterone (HRT) are still considered the most effective treatments for hot flashes and vaginal dryness for most women. Estrogen or HRT can be used if no other treatments are effective or tolerated for menopause symptoms, but should be used with caution and careful follow-up, including yearly mammograms and regular physician evaluations.

For Prevention of Coronary Heart Disease (CHD)
(in women with a history of heart disease)
- estrogen-progesterone therapy *not* recommended

For Treatment of Osteoporosis
- Estrogen or HRT (combined estrogen plus progesterone) is not recommended for routine use at menopause for the prevention or treatment of osteoporosis

For Prevention of Osteoporosis
- estrogen-progesterone or estrogen are *not* recommended as first-line therapy

Whether you use hormone replacement therapy or not is an important decision that should be made by you and your doctor after reviewing your individual risk factors and concerns. Some women prefer long-term therapy with estrogen or estrogen plus progesterone with the full understanding of the benefits and risks as we now know them. For example, it may be appropriate for women who have intolerable symptoms of menopause without the treatment or for women who cannot tolerate other medications currently available for treatment and prevention of osteopenia and osteoporosis.

The FDA now recommends that women who use hormone therapy to manage menopausal symptoms use the lowest effective dose for the shortest amount of time. Some women in our practice continue to take estrogen or estrogen plus progesterone for short-term treatment of symptoms of menopause (usually considered to be less than four or five years). If their gynecologist agrees, some women may take a low-dose oral contraceptive when symptoms of menopause are bothersome between ages forty and fifty. It's important to note that the hot flashes of menopause can worsen if you stop hormonal therapy abruptly. Instead, experts suggest decreasing by one pill a week over six weeks.

Also, if you take short-term estrogen or hormone replacement therapy for menopausal symptoms, the benefits for bone health might disappear after use is discontinued. Studies show that using estrogen for three to five years to relieve symptoms of menopause did very little to prevent fractures from osteoporosis in women when they reached age seventy-five or older. These studies suggested that women who take estrogen to maintain bone density must continue taking estrogen to benefit from its effects on bone health. When estrogen treatment is stopped, bone loss is rapid, just as it is at the time of menopause.

Dr. Laura: "We tell all our patients that no matter what their age they can take steps to prevent bone loss. But the younger you start prevention measures, the better off you'll be. In fact, it's best to build strong bones during childhood and early adulthood, while bone density is naturally increasing, and then continue to strengthen your bones throughout your lifetime. I know that when I'm pushing Bennett's stroller on our evening run I'm doing something good for me—for my present and future bone health."

Use an Integrative Medicine Approach

When we told forty-one-year-old Jessica that she was in perimenopause, the period of about ten years that precedes menopause, she was stunned. Jessica's mother and grandmother had both suffered fractures from osteoporosis before age fifty, so it was even more important for Jessica to evaluate her risk factors for osteopenia. As we emphasized, all women should focus on their risk factors for osteopenia years before menopause to ensure stronger bones after menopause. (Remember, you treat hypertension and high cholesterol years earlier to prevent stroke and heart attack—not after they happen!)

There are safe alternatives to hormone replacement therapy for keeping bones strong—before, during, and after menopause. Integrative medicine therapies incorporate the safest and most effective combinations of natural supplements and bone-boosting medications and are fully discussed in this step.

To Supplement or Not?

The recommended daily allowances (RDAs) are established by the National Academy of Sciences and National Research Council as the amounts necessary to prevent gross deficiency syndromes. It has become apparent to many experts that these levels are not adequate for all people, especially for those with a history of low-calorie dieting or people with chronic diseases. Deprivation dieting can put you at higher risk for nutrient deficiencies as you ingest lower levels of vitamins and minerals. Medications prescribed for chronic illness often wreak havoc with the body. For example, some of our arthritis patients show deficiencies in vitamin C, vitamin D, vitamin E, calcium, and folic acid. Likewise, those patients with osteoporosis are sometimes deficient in vitamin D and calcium. Those who take corticosteroids for any medical problem should consider calcium supplements and other protective medications to make sure they will not suffer bone loss—a side effect of long-term steroid treatment.

If you need supplementation in your diet, follow these safe suggestions:

1. Start with a multiple vitamin that has the Recommended Daily Allowance (RDA) as suggested by the American Dietetic Association.
2. Consult a registered dietitian (R.D.) about your specific vitamin and mineral needs. An R.D. should take into consideration your age, current health status, and medications.
3. Ask your doctor to recommend a safe vitamin-mineral supplement, keeping in mind that a vitamin-mineral supplement should be just that—a supplement to a regular, healthy diet.

In our clinic, we recommend the following integrative medicine approach to reversing osteopenia and preventing fractures:

1. Start with calcium and vitamin D.
2. Know when to add a bone-boosting medication.
3. Consider safe natural dietary supplements.

Different Types of Supplements

- *Time-released* supplements dissolve slowly in the intestine over a 6- to 12-hour period, thus increasing the absorption of a vitamin or mineral.
- *Chelated* minerals are designed to increase absorption in the body.
- *Superpotency* or *therapeutic* supplements contain at least one ingredient in a dose ten times or more greater than the DV (Daily Value).

Start with Calcium and Vitamin D

Along with knowing your risk factors for osteopenia and checking your bone density, regular weight-bearing and strengthening exercises are vital to keep bones strong. You also should make sure you're getting 1,200 to 1,500 mg of calcium and 400 to 1,000 mg of vitamin D each day. (Check the charts on pages 62 and 65 to see how much calcium and vitamin D you need for your age and life stage.)

Ideally, you should get these bone-boosting nutrients through whole foods. However, if your diet does not supply adequate nutrients, we strongly urge you to consider adding natural dietary supplements. Most vitamin-mineral supplements contain 400 mg of vitamin D. In addition, about 15 minutes of sun exposure each day generally allows the body to produce sufficient stores of vitamin D. Adults who work indoors and older adults, especially those in nursing homes, may not get enough sun exposure for adequate vitamin D production. Check with your doctor to make sure your source of vitamin D is adequate.

Assessing Calcium Supplements

Contrary to advertising claims, calcium supplements are *not* all the same. And not all the calcium you eat is absorbed by your body. How much your body absorbs depends on several factors, including the type of calcium compound you take, whether you take it with food or not, and the actual dosage.

You may be wondering, "Why can't I just pop a few antacid tablets in my morning coffee?" Because that might not be the best way to build those bones! Studies have found that not only is the type of calcium important for maximum absorption and bone building, timing and the food you eat or drink with it might be equally important.

For example, if you are a forty-year-old premenopausal woman who needs at least 1,200 mg of calcium each day and take the entire dose at breakfast, research has shown that not all of it will be efficiently absorbed. Also, did you know that if your calcium carbonate tablets contain 500 mg of calcium carbonate, only 200 mg are actually taken in by the body? (See Table 5.1 on page 101.) This means that if you were taking two calcium carbonate antacids each morning, thinking you were getting a full day's requirement, you need to think again. You would need to take six standard (Tums Extra = 500) antacids each day to receive the suggested 1,200 mg. Another tip: calcium carbonate must be taken with food for it to absorb and be used. Popping two antacids of calcium carbonate with coffee is no insurance against serious bone loss.

Be a Discerning Consumer
Are there any rules on calcium supplementation? Calcium advertisements on television and in magazines often confuse the consumer as each claims to be the best way to build strong bones. Grocery and drugstore shelves may add to this confusion, filled as they are with myriad calcium supplements, from calcium carbonate to calcium citrate to calcium phosphate. Not only do the supplements vary, so does the cost. A generic brand might offer the same bone protection as an outrageously priced name brand containing the same ingredient.

In many studies, calcium citrate has been found to dissolve easier than calcium carbonate or calcium phosphate. Researchers state that this form is about 60 percent more *bioavailable*, which means your body can use more of it and gain more benefit. Calcium carbonate and calcium phosphate must be taken with food, but calcium citrate can be taken with or without food. This form of calcium usually does not cause gas and constipation, and you'll find it's more expensive than the other types.

While most nutritionists recommend getting daily calcium through food sources such as dairy products, sardines, or vegetables, some studies have found that the absorption of calcium from calcium carbonate supplements was at least as good as it is from milk. In the research, the supplements contained 400 mg of calcium each (the equivalent of two 500 mg calcium carbonate antacids or four cups of milk) and were taken three times each day—breakfast, lunch, and dinner—for a daily total of 1,200 mg.

Coral Calcium: Truth or Hype?

Coral calcium is a natural dietary supplement that is said to be derived from the dead remains of living coral reefs near Japan. The makers of coral calcium claim that the body will absorb at least twenty times more of this type of calcium than other supplements. They also tout coral calcium as the "cure" for what ails you—osteoporosis, diabetes, cancer, and a host of other chronic illnesses. The truth is there's little proof for any of these claims.

---

8 Ways to Get the Most out of Your Calcium Supplement

1. Instead of taking your entire calcium requirement at one time, divide your calcium into three doses and take with meals throughout the day. The higher the dose taken at one time, the less calcium absorbed by the body.
2. Select chewable or liquid calcium supplements. They are broken down before they enter the stomach and dissolve better in the system.
3. Take most calcium supplements with food; take calcium citrate anytime during the day.
4. Calcium carbonate is the least expensive supplement. It supplies the highest percentage of elemental calcium by weight. Calcium carbonate needs stomach acid to dissolve, so take at the end of a meal. A common—and inexpensive—form of calcium carbonate is found in the antacid Tums and similar products.
5. The market for calcium supplements is huge, and slick manufacturers will say anything to get you to try their product. Be discerning, and choose supplements from reputable companies. Choose calcium supplements of known brand names that have proven reliability. Look for labels that state "purified" or have the USP (United

Table 5.1 Commonly Used Calcium Supplements

Just because you take 1,200 mg of calcium supplementation does not mean your body absorbs 1,200 mg. Review the following table to see the actual amount of calcium the body absorbs with each particular type.

Name	Type of calcium/mg per tablet	Actual amount of calcium absorbed per tablet
Tums tablets	Calcium carbonate 500 mg/tablet	200 mg/tablet
Tums E-X tablets	Calcium carbonate 750 mg/tablet	300 mg/tablet
Tums Ultra	Calcium carbonate 1,000 mg/tablet	400 mg/tablet
Digel tablets	Calcium carbonate 280 mg/tablet	112 mg/tablet
Alkamints tablets	Calcium carbonate 850 mg/tablet	340 mg/tablet
Biocal calcium supplemental tablets	Calcium carbonate 1,250 mg/tablet	500 mg/tablet
Biocal calcium supplemental chewables	Calcium carbonate 625 mg/tablet	250 mg/tablet
Calcium carbonate tablets, generic	Calcium carbonate 500 mg/tablet	200 mg/tablet
Calcium carbonate oral suspension	Calcium carbonate 1,250 mg/tsp	500 mg/tsp
Cal-Sup tablets	Calcium carbonate 750 mg/tablet	300 mg/tablet
Calcium gluconate tablets, generic	Calcium gluconate 500 mg/tablet	45 mg/tablet
Calcium lactate tablets, generic	Calcium lactate 650 mg/tablet	84.5 mg/tablet
Titralac tablets	Calcium carbonate 420 mg/tablet	168 mg/tablet
Caltrate 600	Calcium carbonate 600 mg/tablet	200 mg/tablet
Viactiv	Calcium carbonate 500 mg/tablet	250 mg/tablet
Citracal	Calcium citrate 630 mg/tablet	130 mg/tablet
Oscal Ultra	Calcium carbonate 600 mg/tablet	240 mg/tablet

States Pharmacopeia) symbol. The USP is an independent non-profit organization that sets public quality standards for prescriptions, over-the-counter medications, dietary supplements, and other products. This mark on the product's label signifies that the USP has tested and verified the ingredients, product, and manufacturing process.

6. Avoid calcium from unrefined oyster shell, bone meal, or dolomite without the USP (United States Pharmacopeia) symbol. These have been found to contain higher lead levels.

7. Sometimes calcium supplements can interact with other medications or supplements. For instance, calcium inhibits iron absorption, so don't take your calcium supplement at the same time as an iron supplement. Don't take any medication that requires taking on an empty stomach with a calcium supplement. Talk to your doctor or pharmacist about possible interactions between the other medications and supplements you take.

8. Make sure your calcium supplement is absorbed by your body. To see how well your calcium tablet is absorbed, place it in 3 to 4 ounces warm water or white vinegar for 30 minutes; stir occasionally. If the tablet isn't absorbed in 30 minutes, it probably won't dissolve in your stomach, either.

Know When to Add a Bone-Boosting Medication

If you are one of the millions of women who have osteopenia, you should carefully consider all the facts before you decide whether or not to add medications. If you start a bone-boosting medication, you should expect to take it for a number of years to see optimal results and prevent fractures. Because medication will add to your health care expenses and carries the risk of side effects, it needs to prevent fractures to be worth it.

Even experts don't all agree about when to start medications for osteopenia. Some point to the fact that prevention must start early, just as with hypertension or managing high cholesterol. Others say that until we have more proof that early treatment actually prevents fractures, there's no reason to medicate this large group of people.

But very strong evidence exists that many fractures in postmenopausal women actually happen when bone mass is in the osteopenia range. Some studies show that many fractures (as many as 50 percent or more) actually happen when T scores show osteopenia, not osteoporosis. In other words, a large portion of fractures actually occurs before osteoporosis is present. In addition, there is evidence that medications do lower the risk for fracture in postmenopausal women who have osteopenia—before osteoporosis is labeled.

We might miss the chance to prevent a large number of fractures if we only treat older people with T scores showing osteoporosis. And it is known that those people who have one fracture are at much higher risk of a second fracture. For example, researchers have found that if someone has a fracture in the spine from osteoporosis, there is a greater risk of another spine fracture within a year, along with a higher risk of hip fracture. One in five will have a repeat spine fracture. Why wait for the first fracture?

In our clinical practice we've found that if a woman has osteopenia plus other risk factors present, it is often a good idea to add medication as part of her fracture prevention program. When making the decision as to which medication to use, we always consider factors such as a woman's age, personal health concerns, individual needs, the cost of the medication, and type of insurance, among other things.

Following are a few patient studies indicating the need for medication.

Emme, a thirty-seven-year-old public relations professional, thrives on vigorous exercise—what some might call an exercise obsession. Because of a stressful career, she works out daily at a local fitness center—sometimes twice a day—and takes pride in wearing a size 2. Emme also smokes to suppress her appetite, so she can keep her weight under 120 pounds, and has suffered from loss of menstrual periods (amenorrhea) for the past three years.

However, when her grandmother died after a hip fracture, she decided to have her bone density tested to see if she was at risk for fractures. Here are Emme's risk factors for osteopenia:

1. Exercise obsession
2. Amenorrhea (loss of menstrual periods)
3. Low body weight (below 127 pounds)
4. Smoker
5. Family history of osteoporosis and fractures

Emme's T score was −1.6, indicating osteopenia. Because of her strong family history and personal risk factors, including the female athlete triad (page 3), she was at increased risk for fractures. We started

Emme on Actonel, a medication discussed on page 109 that can build bone density. We will continue to check Emme's T score every two years to see if there is a change. Emme also made a personal commitment to add calcium-rich foods to her diet, reduce her exercise regimen until she regained her menstrual periods, take supplemental calcium, and stop smoking. Her grandmother's hip fracture and death alerted her to the travesty of bone loss and she wants to make changes now, when it can make a big difference.

Forty-nine-year-old Joanne has been postmenopausal for two years. This single woman works part-time as a secretary and also takes care of her invalid mother, who has had three fractures from osteoporosis. Joanne smokes two packs of cigarettes daily and shuns exercise in the humid Florida climate. Here are her risk factors for osteopenia:

1. Postmenopausal
2. Smokes
3. Sedentary lifestyle
4. A family history of osteoporosis and fractures

Joanne had a bone density test a year ago with a T score of −1.2. Her recent bone density test showed a T score of −1.6. Although she didn't have osteoporosis, she did have many risk factors for the disease, and her lower T score showed a possible early warning sign for fractures. We added the medication Fosamax (alendronate) to Joanne's fracture prevention program and now assess her bone mass with a DEXA test every one to two years to make sure the medication is doing its job.

Karin, age fifty-one, is menopausal and has been off hormone replacement therapy for more than six months. This active tennis player fractured her wrist last year, which increases her chance of having another fracture. Here are her risk factors for osteopenia:

1. Menopausal
2. Does not take hormone replacement therapy
3. Wrist fracture

Karin's T score was −1.6, which indicates osteopenia. Because she had an early fracture and had gone off HRT, which can cause faster bone loss (much like a natural menopause), we recommended that Karin start taking Actonel (risedronate), a medication that increases bone density. We will assess her bone mass every one to two years to see if the medication is working.

Gloria, age fifty-three, is postmenopausal and has smoked cigarettes since she was a teenager. This elementary school teacher also takes prednisone for rheumatoid arthritis, an inflammatory arthritis that causes pain, swelling, and stiffness in the joints. It is most common in young women, although it attacks both sexes and all ages. Prednisone greatly increases the risk of osteoporosis and fractures. Here are Gloria's risk factors:

1. Postmenopausal
2. Longtime smoker
3. Takes prednisone, a medication known to decrease bone density
4. Rheumatoid arthritis

Gloria's bone density test's T score was −1.4, which indicated osteopenia. While we don't normally prescribe medication for women with this T score, because of her other risk factors she started taking Fosamax, a bone-strengthening medication. This will help Gloria avoid osteoporosis and fractures.

Jay is a thirty-eight-year-old high school history teacher with rheumatoid arthritis. This young woman has always experienced irregular menstrual periods and has a strong family history of fractures. Because the rheumatoid arthritis is often painful during flareups, Jay has been sedentary over the past few years and does the best she can to work full-time and manage her family.

Here are Jay's risk factors for osteopenia:

1. Rheumatoid arthritis
2. Medications taken to treat the rheumatoid arthritis
3. Irregular menstrual periods
4. Family history of fractures
5. Sedentary lifestyle

Jay's T score was −1.7, indicating osteopenia. Because of Jay's family history and the medications used to treat her rheumatoid arthritis, we recommended that she start taking one of the bone-building medications known to improve bone density and help prevent fractures (see page 109). Jay has increased her calcium intake and is working with a physical therapist to find bone-building exercises that she can do without discomfort. We will assess her bone density annually to make sure this medication is working to increase bone density and to help Jay avoid problems with fractures.

Review the risk factors in the patient stories above. If you have more than one or two risk factors for osteopenia, talk to your doctor. Let your doctor evaluate your health history, perform a bone density test, and then assess your risk factors to see if you might need a bone-strengthening medication to prevent that first fracture. Here are some criteria on which we base our prevention and treatment plan:

T score Indicates Osteopenia (below −1.0 but higher than −2.5)

If you are younger than fifty, and your T score shows osteopenia but you have no other risk factors, talk with your doctor to see if your fracture risk is higher than normal. It's very important that you start Steps 1–3 of the *Bone-Building Program* now, and then repeat the bone density test in one year. If your T score improves (or if it does not drop), then talk with your doctor and decide whether to wait another year before considering medication. If the T score worsens the next year, you may have good reason to consider adding medication to prevent the first fracture.

In many cases, it may not be so obvious that you need to add medication. When you talk to your treating doctor or osteoporosis specialist, consider your T score along with your age and other risk factors—then weigh the possible benefits as well as the cost and risks that would be added along with medication.

If your choice is to be proactive and to do everything you can to prevent the first fracture, you may want to add medication, understanding that you would need to continue for at least a few years before you could judge the results. Or, you can take a more natural approach and follow Steps 1–3 of this program, and then repeat the bone density test in a year.

T score Indicates Osteoporosis (below −2.5)

If your T score is in the osteoporosis range then your risk of fracture is higher and you must start Steps 1–3. You should also talk to your doctor, because you can benefit greatly from adding medication. If you and your doctor decide that the medication may lower your risk of fracture (especially if you have already suffered a fracture), then there are a number of good choices available. These medications should be continued along with the *Bone-Building Program*. Your doctor can also help assess whether other bone-depleting medical problems need treatment.

After one to two years, have a repeat bone density test. With the most commonly used bone-strengthening medications, such as Actonel (risedronate) or Fosamax (alendronate), more than 95 percent of patients respond with an *increase* in bone density measurement in this period of time. In fact, if the bone density drops while taking one of these medications, it's important that your doctor search for another cause to explain the lower score, such as missing medication doses or the development of another medical problem. Medications commonly used to treat osteoporosis are listed on page 109.

Fracture Facts

As you and your doctor decide whether to add a bone-building medication, consider the following fracture facts:

- Early treatment that builds bone has a much better chance of maintaining the original bone strength. Researchers have shown that while osteoporosis patients can increase bone mass, the new mass is not as strong as the original bone.
- It has been shown that many fractures happen in women with osteopenia, before they have osteoporosis measured by bone density test.
- After the first fracture, your risk of more fractures goes up.
- Research shows that if treatment were limited to those who have osteoporosis as indicated by bone density testing (T score of −2.5 or less), most fractures, including many hip fractures, would be missed.
- Studies show that treating people with T score results between −1 and −2.5 does prevent fractures.
- It takes a few years to judge the effectiveness of bone-building medications.

Table 5.2 Help in Making the Medication Decision

Risk Factors	T Score	Diagnosis	Action to Take	Bone Density Test
Age 35–50	−1.0 or higher	Normal	Steps 1–5 for prevention	Repeat in 2 years.
Age 35–50; no risk factors	Between −1.0 and −2.5	Osteopenia	Steps 1–5; talk to your doctor.	Repeat bone density test in 1 year; evaluate.
Age 35–50; previous fracture	−1.7	Osteopenia	Steps 1–5; Talk about medications with your doctor and look at the facts about fractures on page 107.	Repeat bone density test in 1 year if you're taking medication. If you're not taking medication and your score is not improved, talk to your doctor.
• Age 50 and higher	−1.0 or higher	Normal	Steps 1–5 for prevention	Repeat in 2 years.
Age 50 and higher; no other risk factors	−1.3	Osteopenia with no other risk factors	Steps 1–5 for prevention	Repeat in 2 years if you have two risk factors
Age 50 and higher; low body weight; smoker	−1.5	Osteopenia with other risk factors	Steps 1–5 for prevention; discuss medications with your doctor and look at the facts on page 107.	Repeat in 1–2 years on medication. Repeat in 1 year if no medication
Age 50 and higher	−2.0	Osteopenia	Steps 1–5; discuss medication with your doctor after you review the facts on fractures.	Repeat in 1 year.
Age 50 and higher	−2.5	Osteoporosis	Steps 1–5; consider adding bone-building medication after reviewing the facts about fractures.	Repeat in 1–2 years.

Effective Medications for Treating Bone Loss

Your doctor says you are at high risk of fractures. Now what? You should consider taking one of several excellent new medications that help to prevent and treat bone loss. While there is no cure for osteoporosis, some medications can help prevent it, slow it down, or stop and reverse its progress altogether. Because bone density is strongly connected to an increased risk for fractures, we know that as bone density improves, the risk of fractures drops.

Most of the medications described below are proven to increase bone density and lower the risk of fractures. Some have also been proven to lower the risk of fractures in the spine and the hip. Many studies on the effectiveness of these medications have been done in postmenopausal women. Some of the studies were also done in men and in patients taking cortisone medications, which greatly increase the risk of osteoporosis. The risk of fractures dropped over six to twelve months. Many researchers believe that the quick improvement in fracture risk is due to microscopic changes in the structure of the bones that makes them stronger and less likely to break. These microscopic changes happen in addition to the improvement of the total amount of bone present.

The most effective medications to prevent fractures are listed below. These medications have been used mainly in postmenopausal women, but are being used as well in men with osteoporosis, in men and women who take prednisone, and in some perimenopausal women. Your doctor can help you decide whether any of them are appropriate for you.

- **Actonel** (risedronate) is a bisphosphonate, a group of medications that reduces the activity of cells that cause bone loss, to produce a net increase in bone density. Unlike estrogen, the bisphosphonates are not hormones. Instead, bisphosphonates build overall bone mass by slowing the removal of bone while allowing more bone to continue to be formed. Over 95 percent of those treated with bisphosphonates increase their scores on bone density testing.

  Actonel in particular has been shown to lower the risk of spinal fractures by up to 69 percent in one year. In clinical trials, Actonel decreased the chance of spinal fractures in patients taking cortisone medications by 70 percent in one year. It also reduced the risk of hip fractures in women with osteoporosis by about 60 percent after three years.

- **Fosamax** (alendronate) is also a bisphosphonate. In clinical trials of postmenopausal women with osteoporosis, Fosamax reduced bone loss and increased bone density in both the spine and the hip. Fosamax also reduced the risk of spine fractures by up to 62 percent at two years and hip fractures by 56 percent at four years.

  Fosamax and Actonel are usually taken once a week, but can also be taken daily. Once you are up for good in the morning, take it with a 6- or 8-ounce glass of water. Orange juice or coffee can decrease the amount of medication absorbed. It's important not to lie down for 30 to 60 minutes after taking Fosamax or Actonel. After that time you can drink or eat. This usually prevents any symptoms of esophageal irritation such as indigestion, heartburn, or abdominal discomfort.

  Most people do not have problems taking one of these medications, but potential side effects include heartburn, indigestion, or abdominal discomfort; muscle, bone, or joint soreness or aches; other problems such as nausea, vomiting, diarrhea, or constipation are uncommon. If you already have an esophageal problem, especially a narrowing of the esophagus (esophageal stricture), check with your doctor before you take one of these medications.

- **Evista** (raloxifene) is a selective estrogen receptor modulator (SERM) used to build bone in those with osteoporosis. Raloxifene is an anti-estrogen, meaning it blocks the effect of estrogens in breast cancer. The advantage of Evista is that it doesn't increase the risk of breast cancer, which is one reason women are now stopping HRT as a preventive measure against bone loss. Evista also does not cause uterine bleeding, which often occurs with hormone replacement therapy. SERMs are not estrogens, but they have estrogen-like effects on some tissues and anti-estrogen effects on other tissues. Evista has been shown to prevent bone loss, improve the score on bone density testing, and reduce the risk of spine fractures by 30 to 50 percent. It is taken as a tablet once a day.

  Most women tolerate Evista without problems, but potential side effects include hot flashes, clot formation in some blood vessels, muscle soreness, weight gain, or a rash.

- **Miacalcin** (nasal calcitonin) and **Calcimar** (calcitonin) are approved for the treatment of osteoporosis in women who are at least five years beyond menopause. Calcitonin is a hormone (but not an estrogen) that's involved in calcium regulation and bone metabolism. It is usually taken as a single daily nasal spray (Miacalcin) or sometimes as an injection under the skin (Calcimar). In postmenopausal women, calcitonin increases bone density, particularly in the spine. Some have found that Miacalcin (the nasal spray) increased bone density, especially in the first year, but had less effect in the second year of treatment. Studies have shown that Miacalcin lowered the risk of fractures in the spine by 36 percent.

Some patients find that calcitonin also helps relieve pain from spinal fractures.

The most common side effects reported with Miacalcin nasal spray are a runny nose and other signs of nasal irritation. Potential side effects of calcitonin include flushing of the face and hands, increased urinary frequency, nausea, and skin rash.

- **Forteo** (teriparitide) is a synthetic version of *parathyroid hormone*, which is naturally produced in the body and stimulates bone formation. It actually builds new bone by increasing the activity and number of bone-forming cells called *osteoblasts.* All other approved osteoporosis treatments, including Fosamax, Actonel, Evista, Miacalcin, and estrogen, are *antiresorptive*—that is, they slow the rate of bone loss by interfering with bone-destroying cells called *osteoclasts.*

  In clinical trials, Forteo reduced the risk of spinal fractures by 65 percent at nineteen months. This medication is used in patients who have osteoporosis with a high risk of fractures, or for patients with osteoporosis who have failed to respond to or experienced side effects with other medications. It is given as a subcutaneous injection daily.

  The most common side effects of Forteo are dizziness and leg cramps. It is not given for more than two years. Persons who have had Paget's disease (a disease of the bone), radiation treatment to bones, bone cancer, or high blood calcium levels should not take Forteo. As always, talk with your doctor about the benefits and risks of Forteo (or any treatment) to prevent fractures from osteoporosis.

Effective Medications to Build Bone

Brand Name	Generic Name	How Administered
Actonel	risedronate	weekly tablet
Fosamax	alendronate	weekly tablet
Evista	raloxifene	daily tablet
Miacalcin	calcitonin nasal spray	daily nose spray
Forteo	teriparitide	daily injection
Prempro	estrogen plus progesterone	daily tablet
Premarin	estrogen (alone)	daily tablet

> ### Future Thoughts
>
> Scientists are working on a shot given once a year—as opposed to a pill—which researchers believe may be enough to prevent osteoporosis and painful fractures. A study, reported in the February 28, 2002, issue of the *New England Journal of Medicine,* describes a drug called Zometa (zoledronic acid), a bisphosphonate, which is given to cancer patients to treat problems in which calcium leaches from the bones. If subsequent studies are conclusive, men and women might get an annual osteoporosis shot—just as they get their yearly flu vaccine.

Consider Safe Natural Dietary Supplements

Interest in natural therapies to use at menopause is dramatically increasing, especially after the negative findings about hormone replacement therapy. A decade ago, the most popular natural dietary supplement was a vitamin-mineral supplement. Herbal ingredients were scarce, and most people hadn't heard of isoflavones or black cohosh. Today in the United States, dietary supplements include a wide assortment of products, including multivitamins, minerals, amino acids, herbs, as well as ingredients derived from plant and animal sources. These are available in an assortment of forms from capsules, pills, and gel tabs, to liquids, tinctures, extracts, and powders.

While the dietary supplement industry is not regulated by the Food and Drug Administration (FDA), in 1994 the FDA established standards for manufacturers to assure that supplements bear ingredient and nutritional labeling. For instance, according to the FDA, herbal supplements must state the part of the plant from which the ingredient is derived. An herbal supplement such as black cohosh, commonly taken by women to decrease symptoms of menopause, might state on the label "Black Cohosh extract (root) containing 2.5 percent Triterpene Glycosides . . . 160 mg (milligrams). Other ingredients: Rice Powder, Silicon Dioxide, Magnesium Stearate, Gelatin." Other than that, manufacturers are free to make whatever claims they want on the supplement label or in literature, without clinical studies to support them.

If you choose to take a natural dietary supplement, talk to your doctor. Especially if you are taking any medication, you need to make sure the supplement is safe and that there are no medication/supplement interactions that could be harmful to your health.

About Dietary Supplements

Dietary supplements were defined in a law passed by Congress in 1994. According to the Food and Drug Administration (FDA), a dietary supplement must meet all of the following conditions:

- It is a product (other than tobacco) intended to supplement the diet, which contains one or more of the following: vitamins, minerals, herbs or other botanicals, amino acids, or any combination of the above ingredients.
- It is intended to be taken in tablet, capsule, powder, soft gel, gel caplets, or liquid form.
- It is not represented for use as a conventional food or as a sole item of a meal or the diet.
- It is labeled as a dietary supplement.

Phytoestrogens

As discussed on page 69, *phytoestrogens* are plant-based compounds found in certain seeds, nuts, herbs, and fruits that bind to estrogen receptors in the body. It is thought that phytoestrogens give some of estrogen's beneficial effects without the deleterious risks. Perhaps the most common source of phytoestrogens is the isoflavones available in soybeans.

Phytoestrogens are adaptogenic. That is, they tend to suppress estrogen function when it is too high, and supplement estrogen when it is too low. Soy products are a great source of beneficial phytoestrogens. In a study on postmenopausal women who weren't taking hormone replacement therapy, the group who received the most isoflavones (from soy) increased their bone density by 3 percent. In another study, published December 8, 2001, in the *American Journal of Clinical Nutrition*, researchers had perimenopausal women supplement their diets with soy. The research suggested that isoflavones decreased bone loss from the spine in perimenopausal women who were estrogen-deficient. Women like those in this study may be expected to lose bone at an annual rate of 1 to 3 percent per year if they do not take precautions like Steps 1–5 in the *Bone-Building Program*.

In yet another clinical review on the health benefits of phytoestrogens, it was found that rates of heart disease, various cancers, fractures from osteoporosis, and menopausal symptoms are lower among populations that consume plant-based diets, particularly among cultures with diets that are traditionally high in soy products.

Perhaps one of the most convincing studies on isoflavones and bone health comes from Japan. In the study, led by Dr. Yoshiaki Somekawa, women in both the early and late postmenopausal periods who consumed the highest level of isoflavones in foods such as tofu, boiled soybeans, and soy milk, had significantly thicker bones than women who consumed the lowest level of isoflavones. Women in the early postmenopausal period also had significantly fewer backaches and aching joints. Ipriflavone, a synthetic phytoestrogen marketed in Japan and Europe for the prevention and treatment of osteoporosis, is also under active study.

While we still don't know the outcome of taking isoflavone or ipriflavone supplements, we do know there are some positive health benefits from adding soy foods to the diet, as discussed in Step 3. In fact, there are more than 100 protective compounds in soy that can help to boost optimal health. Try to include two servings of soy milk, tofu, or soy-based products in your daily diet if possible.

Fast Facts

40 million	Number of menopausal women in America
5,500	Number of women who enter menopause each day
80.05	Average life expectancy of a woman in 2003
50	Average life expectancy of a woman in the early 1900s
51	Average age of a woman at menopause
10	Average number of years women experience perimenopause

Other Natural Products to Ease Menopausal Symptoms

Without HRT to ease menopausal symptoms, many of our patients tell us they use natural products. The following are popular alternatives for hormone replacement therapy. While some women claim they work to diminish symptoms, the scientific proof and confirmation of long-term safety have not been established.

Black cohosh (Actaea racemosa)
The herb black cohosh contains estrogenic sterols and is widely touted as the cure-all for menopausal symptoms. In several studies comparing black

cohosh with conjugated estrogens and estrogen with progestin, black cohosh provided comparable symptom relief. The herb suppresses the secretion of luteinizing hormone (LH), elevated levels of which are associated with troublesome symptoms. Although it is a phytoestrogen and acts similarly to estrogen, its phytoestrogens are very different from those found in soy products.

In a study published in March 2002 in the *Journal of Women's Health and Gender-Based Medicine,* German researchers funded by the manufacturer of RemiFemin reported on a six-month trial involving 150 peri- and postmenopausal women. Those taking the standard dose of black cohosh (40 mg/day) experienced a 70 percent reduction in symptoms, including hot flashes, mood swings, night sweats, and occasional sleeplessness. Women on a higher dose (127 mg daily) got no additional relief.

The German study also addressed another major concern—whether black cohosh, like estrogen, might increase the risk of certain forms of cancer. The German researchers found that black cohosh did not stimulate changes in vaginal cells or affect levels of several important hormones, including 17-beta estradiol, a form of estrogen.

Even though definitive evidence is not available, a review of current studies indicates that black cohosh is a safe herbal medicine and the most effective botanical for reducing hot flash frequency and intensity. In 2001, the American College of Obstetricians and Gynecologists stated that black cohosh might be helpful in the short term (six months or less) for women with these vasomotor symptoms of menopause.

Although few adverse side effects have been reported with black cohosh, long-term safety data is not available. Women with breast cancer may want to avoid black cohosh until its effects on breast tissue are carefully studied.

Vitamin E

A fat-soluble vitamin and powerful antioxidant, vitamin E may be useful in helping to relieve hot flashes. Antioxidants help to protect cells against the effects of free radicals, which are potentially damaging by-products of the body's metabolism. Free radicals contribute to cell damage, which can result in chronic disease.

In a study published in April 2001 in *The Lancet Oncology,* experts from the Mayo Clinic in Rochester, Minnesota, found that vitamin E, at a dose of 800 international units per day, is modestly effective in reducing hot flashes, cutting the number of hot flashes by one per day. Other drugs, including medications to treat high blood pressure and depression, have shown some effectiveness in treating hot flashes and are being studied further.

Evening primrose (Oenothera biennis)
This botanical is a sweet herb, and contains linoleic acid and gamma-linolenic acid (GLA)—also found in borage seeds and black currant seeds. Linolenic acid is an essential fatty acid (EFA), which means the body does not produce it, so we must replenish our stores with food. Essential fatty acids aid in the production of prostaglandins that counter inflammation. Linolenic acid in particular helps keep skin, vaginal tissue, and other mucous membranes healthy.

EFAs such as linolenic acid (an omega-3 fatty acid) can also be found in fish, flaxseed, pumpkin seed, and walnuts.

Other Natural Products
Some of our patients have asked about progesterone cream, which is sold at health food stores. If you analyze the ingredients in this over-the-counter hormone cream, you'll find it is usually made from wild yams. Although claims are made for the efficacy of this cream, scientific studies do not support its use in easing menopause symptoms or increasing bone density.

A variety of other products have been promoted and sold for menopausal symptoms, including red clover, dong quai, and flaxseed. While there's no evidence that such products are dangerous, neither is there compelling data from clinical trials demonstrating their effectiveness.

Herbs to Induce Relaxation and Sleep

Many women complain of difficulty maintaining sleep during peri-menopause and menopause. If you have difficulty sleeping and want to avoid taking hormones or sleep preparations, one of the following "sleepy-time" herbs might help to increase relaxation and calmness:

Chamomile (Matricaria recutita)
Chamomile depresses the central nervous system and may help relieve anxiety and increase deep sleep. German chamomile is best used as a tea, while Roman chamomile has a bitter taste and is more appropriate as a tincture. Both can be taken in tea or capsules to soothe nerves and induce sleepiness.

Passionflower (Passiflora incarnata)
Passionflower is used as a sedative in Europe and is generally ingested as a tea before bedtime. Passionflower is available as a tea, tincture, in capsules, and extracts. Take near bedtime for a restful night's sleep.

Valerian (Valeriana officinalis)
Valerian is a spicy, bitter herb with sedative properties used to calm the central nervous system, making it useful for treating anxiety, insomnia, and stress. Take valerian in tea, tincture, or capsules about thirty minutes before bedtime to fall asleep easily.

St. John's Wort (Hypericum perforatum)
St. John's wort is another popular choice among midlife women for relieving mild depression without some of the common side effects of prescription antidepressants. While this herb seems safe, check with your doctor before taking it, since symptoms of depression can be serious. St. John's wort should not be used concurrently with antidepressants.

Caution!

Before taking the herbal supplements discussed in this step, talk to your doctor or pharmacist about possible side effects or herb-drug interactions. Herbal therapies are not recommended for pregnant women, children, the elderly, or those with compromised immune systems. In addition, some herbs have sedative or blood-thinning qualities, which may dangerously interact with NSAIDs or other pain medications. Others may cause gastrointestinal upset if taken in large doses.

No herb or pharmaceutical is 100 percent safe and effective. In 2002 some forty people were reported to have died from the misuse of herbs. Still, this number does not begin to approach the percentage of casualties caused by FDA-approved drugs. Whether you're considering a natural dietary supplement or an FDA-approved pharmaceutical, know that there will likely be some side effect, along with the positive healing effect. A good website that keeps consumers informed about dietary supplements that may be unsafe or recalled is www.fda.gov/medwatch/safety.htm. Check this site periodically to ensure any supplements you're taking are safe.

Change Lifestyle Habits to Reverse Osteopenia

As you have read in this step, there is no magic pill to protect your bones from osteopenia and fractures. If there were, then there would be no need for this book! The most effective preventive measure you can take right now—no matter what your age or life stage—is to follow healthy lifestyle practices, including the following:

- Know the risk factors for osteopenia. Don't hesitate to get a bone density test and evaluate your T score with your doctor (Step 1). (Use the chart on page 108 to assess your T score.)
- Increase your weight-bearing and strengthening exercises (Step 2).
- Change your daily diet to include foods high in bone-strengthening nutrients (Step 3).
- Avoid tobacco products and consume alcohol in moderation (Step 4).
- Fall-proof your home (Step 4).
- Talk with your doctor about bone-boosting medications and natural dietary supplements (Step 5).

A painful fracture can dramatically change your life. But it's important to realize that you have a good deal of control over your bone health. We now realize that the connection between low bone density measured on a DEXA test and the risk of fracture is stronger than the connection between hypertension and stroke or between high cholesterol and heart attack. That's why it's important to periodically assess your risk factors for osteopenia and decide about a bone density test. Stay in touch with your doctor if your T score worsens, and learn about bone-boosting medications.

While it's never too late to stop fractures, we believe that it's far better to take the necessary steps early to prevent fractures altogether.

CHAPTER 6

Special Situations

Whether male or female, everyone is at risk for bone loss and fractures unless they are taking active steps to keep bones strong. As discussed in earlier chapters, even college-age women run the risk of measurable bone loss if they fail to recognize telltale risk factors and take action.

In this chapter our aim is to target five different groups of people who need specific recommendations to strengthen bone and prevent bone loss, osteoporosis, and pain from fractures:

1. Children and teens
2. Postmenopausal women
3. Men
4. Those with spinal fractures and back pain
5. Those who need surgery

Special Situation 1: Children and Teens

Ultimately, protection against osteopenia should start in childhood. Although your parents may not have known this, you are now equipped with information and tools to give your kids a bone-boosting advantage with diet and exercise.

Up to 90 percent of peak bone mass is acquired by age eighteen in girls and age twenty in boys, which makes childhood and adolescent years the *best time* for your kids to "invest" in their bone health. Before puberty, boys and girls develop bone mass at similar rates. After puberty, however, boys tend to acquire greater bone mass than girls.

When a girl has her first menstrual period, bone mass is increasing at its highest pace. Yet instead of taking advantage of building bones while the body is primed to do so, reports show that the average teenage girl gets only about 300 to 800 mg of bone-boosting calcium a day. The optimal bone-building requirement for a nine-year-old girl is 1,300 mg or the equivalent of almost five glasses of milk. (See Children's Calcium Guidelines, Table 6.1, below.)

Medications used to treat chronic health problems such as asthma or rheumatoid arthritis may also contribute to a child's risk of early bone loss. Many young patients are treated with prednisone or other cortisone (corticosteroid) derivative medications. Bone loss with these medications is extremely common even in younger people who have no other risk factors for osteopenia. (If your child takes prednisone, talk with your pediatrician to see what additional measures you can take to ensure strong bones during childhood.)

Still, as much as we know about ways to prevent or reverse osteopenia, a new finding reported in the September 2003 issue of the *Journal of the American Medical Association* confirms that there is more work to do. In this study, researchers compared the rate of wrist fractures among young people over the past three decades and found a statistically significant increase of 42 percent in the 1999–2001 period over the 1969–1971 period. This finding of increased fractures suggests impaired bone-mass development, which could spell trouble later in life. It does not have to be this way. Assess your child's risk factors, diet, and exercise habits now— and then make plans to follow our program to build strong bones.

Table 6.1 Children's Calcium Guidelines

Ages	Amount of Calcium
Up to 6 months	210 mg
6 months to 1 year	270 mg
1 to 3 years	500 mg
4 to 8 years	800 mg
9 to 13 years	1,300 mg
14 to 18 years	1,300 mg

*SOURCE: *National Academies' Institute of Medicine (NAIM)*

NOTE: One 8-ounce glass of milk equals about 300 milligrams of calcium.

Be Aware of Risk Factors

Your child's bone mass is influenced by various factors. Some of these factors, such as race or gender, cannot be changed. Other risk factors can be changed, including eating calcium-rich foods and exercising daily.

Gender
Women are at higher risk for bone loss than men. While boys and girls develop bone mass at a comparable pace until puberty, at that time boys start to attain greater bone mass than girls.

Race
African-American girls tend to achieve higher peak bone mass than Caucasian girls do. Consequently, African-American women are at lower risk for developing osteoporosis later in life.

Hormones
The sex hormones estrogen and testosterone are necessary for the development of bone mass. Girls who menstruate at an early age usually have greater bone density than girls who menstruate later. Those who frequently miss their menstrual periods sometimes have lower bone density.

Nutrition
Calcium deficiencies in children and adolescents account for a 5 to 10 percent lower peak bone mass and may contribute to an increased risk for bone fractures later. Children need a bone-building diet, as described in Step 3, with foods high in vitamins C, D, and K, calcium, and trace minerals.

Physical Activity
Physical exercise is vital for building healthy bones. The benefits of activity are most pronounced in those areas of the skeleton that bear the most weight, such as the hips during walking and running and the arms during gymnastics and upper-body weight lifting.

Take Bone-Building Action

There are three simple ways you can protect your child from osteopenia and fractures in later years:

1. Feed those bones.
2. Get daily exercise.
3. Watch for eating disorders.

Feed Those Bones
To prevent osteopenia in later years, your child needs plenty of nutritious foods high in calcium and vitamin D. In an interesting United States Department of Agriculture (USDA) nationwide food consumption survey titled "What We Eat in America," researchers found that on any given day, nearly half of three- to five-year-olds and roughly two-thirds of school-age youth, ages six through nineteen, consumed food or drink outside the home. By the teen years, fast-food restaurants rank highest as the most frequent food source. While there is an upward trend in beverage consumption for children and teens, the biggest increase is in noncitrus juices and soft drinks. Milk consumption, on the other hand, dropped dramatically—only half of today's teens drink milk. Nutritional surveys estimate that as many as 84 percent of teenage girls do not get the necessary 1,300 to 1,500 milligrams of daily calcium needed for bone health. Statistics also show that more than 80 percent of all girls are dieting between the bone formative years of eight and fifteen.

Another intriguing study by the National Institute of Child Health and Human Development concluded that supplementing the diets of girls, ages twelve through sixteen, with 500 mg of calcium daily produced a 14 percent increase in bone density in comparison to unsupplemented girls. The implications of this increase are striking: *for every 5 percent increase in bone density as a child, the risk of fracture later in life declines by 40 percent.*

To Do: Review the dietary information in Step 3 and include bone-building foods in your child's daily diet. Also, include some of the Bone-Building Recipes in chapter 7 in your daily meal plan. These recipes are tasty and will appeal to fussy eaters while helping to keep young bones strong.

To Do: Vitamin D, another key bone-building nutrient discussed on page 63, helps the body absorb calcium. While most kids who play outdoors get plenty of vitamin D, make sure your child also gets vitamin D from fortified milk, tuna fish, or eggs.

Get Daily Exercise
Exercise is also a vital stimulus for developing bones. Some findings even indicate that babies who kick a lot in the womb appear to have stronger bones!

An intriguing study, reported in the December 2003 issue of *Pediatrics*, concluded that regular jumping exercises might delay the onset of bone loss. The two-year study compared 34 girls who took physical education classes three days a week to 46 girls who did not exercise. The participants in the study alternated vigorous jumping exercises with running or skipping. The girls in the study had nearly a 5 percent gain in bone minerals when compared to the girls who did not exercise. Again, from

---

Supplement If Necessary

We believe that whole foods are the best source of bone-building nutrients. But if your child does not get adequate dietary calcium, talk to your family doctor about a calcium supplement. Review the information on page 120, and be sure to give no more than 500 mg of calcium at one time.

---

4 Ways to Get Kids to Move Around More

If your child is sedentary, here are some ways to get her or him to move around more and start building stronger bones:

1. *Move while watching television.* Get your child a jump rope or mini-trampoline, and let her exercise while watching a favorite sitcom.

2. *Walk with your child.* Take time after dinner each night to go for a walk with your child. Don't call it "exercise," but let the child know it's your special time together.

3. *Turn off the video games.* Schedule limited time each day for computer use and video games, then unplug! During the off time, encourage your child to ride a bike, jump rope, or take the family dog for a walk.

4. *Play together.* On weekends, spend time outdoors with your child at a nearby playground. Toss a ball around, Rollerblade, or climb the jungle gym together. During inclement weather, go to a skating rink, bowling alley, or indoor gym and enjoy being physically active with your child. Be sure to include weight-bearing activities such as jumping rope, dancing, climbing stairs, tennis, and volleyball in your playtime. In addition, team sports such as soccer, basketball, softball, and baseball are excellent for stimulating bone growth.

current research findings we know that increasing bone mass during childhood is great protection against bone loss and fractures later in life.

To Do: We believe that almost every child can exercise daily for at least forty-five minutes to an hour or longer. (Remember, kids call this play—not work!) This exercise should include weight-bearing activities, which determine the strength, shape, and mass of bone. Exercises such as walking, jogging, soccer, aerobics, jumping rope, stair climbing, and dancing are all weight-bearing and bone-stimulating. As we discuss on page 123, strength-training activities such as push-ups and climbing the jungle gym also help to keep bones strong.

Your child can receive a great bone benefit from being involved in youth athletics, whether baseball, softball, soccer, or football. If your child is shy or does not care to be part of a large group, you can encourage an individual activity such as ballet, gymnastics, swimming, or crew. Although swimming is not a weight-bearing exercise, it does build strong muscles that support the back.

Exercise Bonus

Regular exercise releases "feel-good" hormones, endorphins. Just thirty minutes of exercise, every other day, can help irritable or moody kids and teens enjoy better moods within two to three weeks.

Watch for Eating Disorders

As you stay on top of your child's eating and exercise habits, be sure to watch for early signs of eating disorders. As discussed on page 55, eating disorders, particularly anorexia nervosa, can lead to early bone loss or osteopenia in young women. Anorexia often causes irregular menstrual periods or the complete absence of periods, known as amenorrhea. The latter is a sign of low estrogen, the hormone necessary for protecting bone density and achieving optimal bone mass.

To Do: Talk to your family doctor if your child shows any of the following signs of an eating disorder:

• Missed menstrual periods after having had them regularly for at least several months

- Extreme and/or unhealthy-looking thinness
- Extreme weight loss
- Eats little food or just plays with food
- Does not eat with the family
- Makes frequent trips to the bathroom after mealtime
- Preoccupied with being thin
- Overtraining or excessive exercise

8 Kid-Friendly Bone-Building Tips

1. Add 2 tablespoons milk powder (400 mg calcium) to a glass of low-fat milk (300 mg calcium). Stir, then freeze in ice-cube trays and use instead of ice cubes for a high calcium boost to milk shakes or tofu smoothies.
2. Make sure your child gets ample vitamin D through 15 to 20 minutes of sun exposure each day and by drinking vitamin D–fortified milk.
3. Add evaporated skim or nonfat milk to your recipes that call for milk to double the calcium intake without doubling the fat calories.
4. Sprinkle almonds or sunflower seeds on salads and casseroles to increase your child's magnesium and phosphorus intake, both vital for bone health.
5. Incorporate soy products at least once a day to increase your child's bone strength. Use soy granules as a filler for meat dishes or vegetable casseroles or substitute tofu in recipes.
6. If a recipe calls for 1 cup milk (300 mg calcium), replace this with calcium-fortified milk (1 cup = 500 mg calcium). If your child is allergic to cows' milk, consider calcium-fortified soy milk or rice milk for cooking (1 cup = 300 mg).
7. Whenever possible, substitute milk for water in a recipe. Milk is composed of 90 percent water, yet it is full of bone-boosting vitamins and minerals.
8. Add calcium-fortified orange juice instead of water to congealed salads (1 cup = 300 mg).

Foods for Stronger Bones

1. Dairy products (such as milk, cheese, cream cheese, yogurt, ice cream, and cottage cheese)
2. Calcium-fortified foods (such as cereals, rice, yogurt, breads, and cottage cheese)
3. Soy products (such as tofu, soybeans, soya granules, soy flour, soy nuts, and miso)
4. Salmon and sardines, fresh or canned
5. Fresh fruits (such as apricots, bananas, cantaloupe, mango, orange, papaya, and strawberries)
6. Spinach, broccoli, collards, kale, and turnip or mustard greens
7. Whole grains, especially those that are calcium-fortified
8. Lentils, seeds, and nuts
9. Green and black tea, especially if made with fluoridated water
10. Egg and egg substitute

Special Situation 2: Postmenopausal Women

We tell all of our patients that the fracture you want to prevent *is the first one*. That's because once you have one fracture, your risk of having more fractures greatly increases. After a spine fracture, about 20 percent of patients may have another fracture within a year. New findings in fact conclude that the risk of a subsequent fracture is highest directly after the first break, which provides strong grounds for intervention immediately after a fracture.

Researchers have shown that up to 50 percent of women in their 50s have either low bone mass or osteoporosis. This increases with age: more than 90 percent of all women in their 80s have osteoporosis. Sadly, less than 1 in 5 older women know about the problem and are being treated with effective medication. Even with all the education over the last few years, most of these women will not find out about bone thinning until the first fracture.

If you are postmenopausal and at higher risk for osteoporosis, if you've already been diagnosed with low bone density, or if you have experienced a fracture, consider some proactive ways to keep your bones strong—so you don't experience fractures in the future. There is a way to stop this decline in bone strength and repetitive fractures: take control now and start the *Bone-Building Program*. Let's look at several patients who did just that:

Nancy's Fractured Ankle

Nancy, an enormously successful fifty-one-year-old retailer, tripped on an uneven sidewalk in front of her shop and suffered a painful broken ankle. This slim Caucasian woman had smoked two packs of cigarettes a day for as long as she could remember. Nancy had a surgical hysterectomy at forty and did not take estrogen therapy. Her career in retail was mostly sedentary, and she admitted that she had not exercised for years.

After the ankle fracture, we did a bone density test that showed Nancy's T score to be −2.9. This score indicated that her risk of future fractures was abnormally high for a woman in her early fifties.

Risk Factors

- Fifty-one-year-old Caucasian female
- Slim build; underweight
- Smoker (two packs a day)
- An early menopause at forty (hysterectomy); no HRT
- A sedentary job; no exercise program
- Bone density spine T score –2.9

Bone-Building Treatment

Nancy immediately began the *Bone-Building Program*, including adding calcium and vitamin D supplements, regular weight-bearing and strengthening exercises, and stopping smoking. She added medication, Fosamax (alendronate, discussed on page 110), which she took weekly. Nancy also changed the shoes she wore to help her feel sturdier when walking and began a tai chi class at a local fitness center to improve her balance and flexibility—all important factors in fall prevention. She plans to have another bone density scan in about one year.

Shirley's Fractured Ribs

Sixty-one-year-old Shirley was being treated for chronic bronchitis. This two-packs-a-day smoker had taken prednisone treatment occasionally for a few weeks at a time over recent years for the bronchitis. Because of her breathing problem, Shirley was uncomfortable exercising and had a sedentary job as an administrative assistant at a law firm.

Over the Christmas holidays, Shirley visited her daughter and young grandchildren. While picking up her two-year-old grandson, she felt a sharp pain in her chest—she'd fractured two ribs. Shirley's daughter brought her to our clinic and she had a bone density scan, which showed her to have a T score of −2.9, or 2.9 standard deviations below normal for her age.

Risk Factors

- Sixty-one-year-old Caucasian female
- Normal weight
- Smoker (two packs a day)
- Chronic obstructive pulmonary disease (COPD); prednisone for twelve years
- A sedentary job; no exercise program
- A history of rib fractures with lifting
- Bone density of hip T score −2.9

Bone-Building Treatment
Shirley was not ready to retire or give up visiting with family and friends and began treatment immediately to avoid more fractures. She increased her calcium and vitamin D supplementation, started exercising under the guidance of a physical therapist, and added a bone-strengthening medication. After one year, Shirley's bone density increased by 4 percent. She is now proactive and taking the steps necessary to avoid fractures altogether.

Anne's Fractured Hip
Seventy-year-old Anne lived alone when she fell and broke her hip. She had been thin most of her adult life, and as a lifelong smoker she suffered from emphysema and took prednisone (a cortisone medication) to control her breathing. Anne had menopause at age forty-six but did not take estrogen therapy and had avoided milk products for most of her life because of an allergy to the protein in dairy products. She said her mother and aunt were both short and stooped over in later years.

After surgery to repair the broken hip, Anne went to a nearby nursing home for physical therapy. While there, she had a bone density test of her good hip with a resulting T score of −3.2.

Risk Factors

- Seventy-year-old Caucasian female
- Small stature; underweight
- Smoker
- COPD (chronic lung disease)—twenty years treated with prednisone
- An early menopause at age forty-six with no estrogen treatment
- Allergy to milk protein (no dairy products)
- Family history
- Bone density non-fractured hip T score −3.2

Bone-Building Treatment

We started Anne on 1,500 milligrams of supplemental calcium and 800 IU of vitamin D each day. She also started taking Actonel (risedronate, see page 109), which is known to increase bone strength and lower the chance of fractures of the hip by about 60 percent. As Anne gained strength, a physical therapist helped her begin the Bone-Building Workout, outlined in Step 2. She started slowly with stretches and range-of-motion exercises (see page 187), and then began walking short distances several times each day. When Anne went home, she continued the dietary supplements and medication, and started a smoking cessation program. She also began a regular exercise program and even joined an exercise class at the local Y.

After one year, Anne's bone density test showed a dramatic increase of 3.5 percent and her T score increased to −2.9. Her risk of fracture was already less, and she was determined to take control of her bone health by staying with the *Bone-Building Program*.

Fractures Take Away Your Independence

Fractures in other locations are more common than the hip fractures Anne had. For example, fractures in the bones of the spine (vertebral fractures) can cause pain in the back, but often may happen without any pain or other sign. If left untreated, they can continue and as more fractures happen, back pain and stooped over posture—a dowager's hump—can be permanent. The curvature of the dowager's hump is a result of the collapse of the spinal column. It is now known that a fracture in the spine also increases the risk of other serious illness, even death.

Those with osteoporosis commonly fracture wrists and shoulders, but a break can happen almost anywhere in the body. A fracture may be the result of an injury, such as one sustained in an auto accident. Moreover, as osteoporosis continues its course, fractures may result from the stress of normal daily activity. Opening a window, simple lifting, or a minor fall can eventually bring on a fracture when the bones are thin. We've seen other patients like Shirley who lifted a young child and fractured a rib. We even have a few patients who suffered a rib fracture during a welcome hug from a friend!

Fractures rob you of an active and independent life. For instance, if a hip fracture or other fractures reduce your ability to do daily activities, you'll have to depend on family and friends to assist you. This loss of independence adds to the stress of the painful fracture. As you become less active, you might feel depressed and withdraw from your social network.

Loss of independence is frightening—and something to avoid if possible. This may be why surveys show that 80 percent of women over age 75 actually prefer death to a hip fracture, which often makes long-term nursing home care necessary.

It does not have to be this way! Using the new testing methods and breakthrough bone-building medications, everyone can enjoy continued mobility, independence, and freedom from pain. You can start the easy steps for treatment and prevention of further problems that will allow you to enjoy an active life. Following are some strategies to prevent fractures from robbing you of an active and independent life:

Fracture Prevention Strategies

Prevention Strategy #1: Review your risk factors for osteoporosis (see below) and talk to your doctor about a bone density test.

Step 1 will help you understand how the bone density test works and what the resulting T score means for your bone health. If you've had a bone density test, review the table on page 108 and follow the specific guidelines for preventing further bone loss. Have a bone density test every one to two years to ensure your bones don't fall into the "danger zone" where they may readily fracture.

Prevention Strategy #2: Follow Steps 2 to 4 in the Bone-Building Program.

It is never too late to protect bones' strength, even though many women begin to experience fractures post menopause because of the decline of estrogen.

Review Step 2 and make a commitment to a consistent exercise

Try Hip Protectors

If you are unsteady when you walk or if you have fallen, consider wearing hip protectors. This lightweight underwear is worn under your dress or slacks and is completely invisible to others. Pockets on each hip accommodate pads that do the real work. The garment doesn't interfere with normal movement but simply gives you extra padding in key areas. Hip protectors lower the chance of hip fracture by 50 percent if you happen to fall.

---

program. Be sure you include weight-bearing exercise (walking or low-impact aerobics), along with strengthening exercises, as discussed on page 35. These work together to stimulate bone-building cells and can help to prevent fractures—no matter what your age. Using a rowing machine or ergometer is an excellent exercise for older women. Rowing builds back muscles, and stronger back muscles mean stronger bones.

In Step 3, we've given the requirements for a bone-building diet. Compare your current eating plan with these recommendations and make plans to add foods high in calcium, vitamins C, D, and K, and the trace minerals (listed on page 58). If you find you cannot get ample calcium (1,500 mg daily), then turn to Step 5 for suggestions on choosing the best calcium supplements. Also, a diet high in soy foods such as tofu, soy milk, and soy by-products has been shown to increase bone strength. Soy foods are high in isoflavones, a plant compound that mimics the effects of estrogen without the deleterious side effects. These foods may help you with menopausal symptoms such as hot flashes if eaten regularly.

Step 4 is crucial for any age, especially as we get older. Preventing falls is one way you can prevent fractures. Follow the guidelines in Step 4 and make sure your home and yard are "fall-proofed." Also, adhere to the specific information on stopping smoking, avoiding excess alcohol consumption, and watching caffeine and cola intake—as all of these can result in decreased bone density.

Prevention Strategy #3: Add calcium and vitamin D supplements to your diet, if necessary.

Unless you are a very healthful eater and include many high-calcium foods in your daily diet, you will need to supplement your intake of this bone-building mineral. Make sure you are now getting 1,500 mg of calcium each day between diet and supplements (see page 98). We find that many postmenopausal women only get from 600 to 800 mg of calcium in their daily diet. In addition, there are studies confirming that 80 percent of all postmenopausal women do not get adequate calcium to stop bone loss.

Vitamin D is also necessary to prevent osteoporosis, and at this life stage, you should be getting 800 IU daily. It is estimated that about fifteen minutes of sun exposure may allow the body to produce vitamin D. If you live in the northern part of the country or work indoors, you will need to make sure your foods are vitamin D fortified or you will need to rely on supplements.

Prevention Strategy #4: Talk to your doctor about your personal need for bone-strengthening medications.

Review the information in Step 5 (page 90) and then discuss your health situation with your personal physician. If you were taking hormone replacement therapy (HRT) or estrogen and have recently stopped, be sure to have a bone density test. Bone loss is as fast after stopping estrogen and HRT as it is at menopause. You can then make specific plans to protect your bones.

The medications listed on page 111 have been found to reverse osteopenia, build bone, and lower the chance of fractures. Talk to your doctor about these medications and ask if any of them could help in your quest to prevent fractures.

Prevention Strategy #5: Educate yourself about medications and illnesses known to increase the risk of osteoporosis and fractures.

We've listed the most common illnesses and medications that can rob you of bone strength. If you have one of these health problems or if you take one of the medications listed, ask your doctor how you can minimize the extra risk brought by the need for certain medications. Usually there are simple steps that can control the added risk. For example, those who take prednisone for asthma and other lung diseases can take medications (see Step 5) to counteract prednisone's bone-thinning effects.

Your Goal: Prevent the First Fracture

If you have experienced menopause—either naturally or as a result of surgery, you need a bone density test. With this information you can plan a prevention strategy years before osteopenia or osteoporosis to prevent the first fracture.

If you haven't had a bone density test, you probably won't be treated with the most effective medications available. Don't hesitate to ask for a bone density test—any more than you would hesitate to have your blood pressure or blood cholesterol tested! Together, you and your doctor can assess your health and lifestyle habits and then put together a personalized *Bone-Building Program* that helps your bones stay strong for the rest of your life.

Special Situation #3: Men, Osteopenia, and Osteoporosis

We wrote this book primarily with younger women in mind, but that doesn't mean men are immune to bone thinning and fractures. Because men have bigger bones to start with, they are less susceptible than women are to bone loss. But they are vulnerable all the same—it just takes a few more years (about ten) for the risks to catch up to them. In fact, of the 40 million at risk for low bone mass and osteoporosis in the United States, about *30 percent are men.*

Estimates from the National Institutes of Health are that about 12 million men have osteoporosis and another 13 million probably have osteopenia. (Although the media has yet to focus on this, the risk of osteoporosis in men is thought to be greater than the risk of prostate cancer.) Still, even fewer men than women know about osteoporosis— what it is, what it can do to the bones, how it is detected, and how it can be prevented and treated. Even though there are effective medications available to prevent fractures, most men are not aware that osteoporosis is a devastating disease that can happen to them.

We know that many healthy living programs for men begin with a caring spouse. It's important that women understand all they can about bone loss in men. Effective treatment, if started early on, can increase bone mass and prevent fractures in men. But we cannot start treatment until a diagnosis is made. Diagnosis starts with a bone density test (see page 19).

We've reviewed studies showing that even after a fracture, most men don't receive bone-strengthening medication to build bone and prevent the next fracture, even though most doctors are aware that after one fracture, the risk of subsequent fractures increases. Researchers have found that even after a hip fracture with hospital treatment and surgery, men who were checked by a physician one year later were usually *not* being treated with medication such as those described in Step 5.

After reading this information, share it with the men in your life and encourage them to read this section.

Bone Loss in Men

Severe bone loss can be just as devastating to men as to women. Among men with hip fractures, 50 percent never fully recover and 25 percent require long-term nursing home care. Hip fractures are the most common reason for admissions to nursing homes. About one-third don't maintain their independence after suffering a hip fracture. But the most serious problem is a higher risk of death—it's even higher in men than in women who have hip fractures. The risk of death in the first year after hip fracture increases with age, and can reach 50 percent by age seventy to eighty. Researchers conclude that elderly men 80 and older actually have a much higher risk of death than women after a hip fracture—*three times more*—although the reasons for the higher risk of death in men aren't clear.

When you add the cost of hip surgery (around $40,000 to $50,000) to these statistics, it makes it worthwhile to look hard at prevention of osteoporosis and fractures altogether.

The elevated risk for low bone mass in men starts after age fifty-five. You might wonder then if all men should have bone density testing at this age. Definitely not. Men who should be concerned about bone health at this age need to read about the risk factors.

Review the following list and discuss with the man in your life to see if he needs to have a bone density test and assess his bone health: some risk factors alone, such as height loss, spine fractures, fractures after age fifty, and cortisone medications, make a bone density test necessary to give the doctor much-needed information. When our male patients have *more than two risk factors*, we recommend a bone density test.

Men with height loss. If you have lost height from your usual adult height, remember that the most common cause is shortening of the bones of the spine (compression fractures) due to osteoporosis. Don't wait until you've lost two or more inches to get your bone density test. Early detection can lead to prevention of future height loss and serious fractures.

Men with spine fractures. Since most spine fractures do not cause any pain, when a fracture is found it is often news to the patient. In fact, spine fractures usually come to our attention when a chest X ray is done as part

Men's Risk Factors for Osteoporosis

Height loss*
Spine fractures*
Any other fracture after age 50*
Cortisone medications*
Age (over 65)
Smokes
Heavy use of alcohol
Chronic lung disease—asthma, chronic bronchitis, emphysema
Family history of osteoporosis
Kidney stones
Low testosterone (male hormone) levels
Severe liver disease
AIDS/HIV and other medical problems

*If you have any of these four risk factors, you need to talk with your doctor soon about a bone density test.

of a routine examination. By far the most common cause of spine fracture is osteoporosis. If your X ray shows you have had a spine fracture, get a bone density test, even if you don't have back pain. This could be a first warning signal and opportunity to take much-needed treatment. The next signal could be a hip fracture or more spine fractures, height loss, and stooped posture.

If you do have back pain, get an X ray, which will indicate if you have had a spine fracture. This may be the earliest warning sign that bone mass is low. If there is a fracture, a bone density test is your next move.

Men with any other fracture after age 50. If you have any other fracture after age fifty, consider a bone density test. If this is the signal that you are developing low bone mass, it could be a great opportunity to treat osteoporosis early when treatment is most effective.

Men with back pain after age 50. If you have back pain, especially if you haven't had an injury or other explanation for the pain, an X ray may reveal a spine fracture at the root of the pain. A bone density test can be done to confirm the diagnosis of osteoporosis. When found early, excellent treatment for osteoporosis is available that can stop future fractures.

After reviewing your risk factors, taking a medical history, and performing an examination, your doctor can determine if an X ray is indicated.

Treatment with cortisone medications. Many health problems such as chronic bronchitis, asthma, emphysema, colitis, and arthritis are successfully treated with prednisone or other cortisone (corticosteroid) derivative medication.

If you have been treated for more than three months with prednisone or a similar drug, or if you require these medicines frequently during the year but not for three months in a row, talk with your doctor about your bone health. You may need to have a bone density test or use a medication to prevent bone loss, which is very common with cortisone medications.

Bone loss with these medications is also extremely common in younger people who have no other risk factors for osteoporosis. If you don't start a preventive medication, you should at least measure your bone density to know where the bone strength stands, and then repeat this test in one year. Most people who are treated with prednisone don't receive additional medication to prevent bone loss—but they should. If you take prednisone, talk with your doctor to see if you should add one of the effective bone-building treatments listed in Step 5.

Age. No one likes to think about getting older, but the risk of low bone mass does increase with age. By age sixty-five, men are at risk for bone loss, which can be found early—before fractures ever occur—with a bone density test. Some experts now recommend bone density testing for *all* men over sixty-five.

Alcohol and smoking. Just as in women, excessive alcohol consumption (more than three drinks per day) and smoking cigarettes can raise the risk of low bone mass. Detecting the problem early allows you to take long-term prevention matters in hand. It may be a good idea to have a bone density test if you are over age fifty and smoke or drink alcohol in excessive amounts.

Other medical problems that cause osteoporosis. In men, a low level of the male hormone testosterone can cause fatigue, loss of sex drive, and other medical problems. Low testosterone, a common cause of low bone mass and osteoporosis, is a condition that can be easily treated with medications.

Family history of osteoporosis. Researchers believe that there may be a genetic risk for bone loss in men, just as there is for women. If you have a family member who suffered fractures such as hip fracture, height loss, or stooped posture, especially in men in your family, discuss bone density testing with your doctor.

Kidney stones. Researchers have found that a man who has had kidney stones may be at higher risk for bone loss as well. The causes are not known, but a study published in the July 2003 issue of the *New England Journal of Medicine* gives evidence that men who have kidney stones should be aware that they may be at higher risk. It may be a good idea to consider a bone density test in many cases.

Other medical problems that can increase the risk of low bone mass and fractures include high or low calcium levels in the blood, severe liver disease, and AIDS/HIV. Your doctor can check your overall health to be sure all systems are working properly and are not contributing to your risk of low bone mass.

Prevention and Treatment

To prevent and treat osteopenia and osteoporosis, men can follow the *Bone-Building Program*, outlined in Steps 1 to 5.

Prevention strategy 1: Be your own bodyguard. Know the risk factors that are specific to men, and ask your doctor for a bone density test if you have more than two of these risk factors. If you have one of the first four risk factors marked with an asterisk (page 135), you should ask your doctor for a bone density test right now.

Prevention strategy 2: Start the Bone-Building Workout. Review the specific types of exercise in this step and make a plan to exercise daily to stimulate your bones to get stronger.

Prevention strategy 3: Make bone-building food choices. Be sure that you are eating plenty of high-calcium foods and other bone-building nutrients. If not, see Step 5 for ways to complement your diet with natural dietary supplements.

Prevention strategy 4: Take strong steps to prevent fractures. Keep your risk of falls low. An exercise program can strengthen the back and legs, helping to make you steadier. Walking also helps to increase strength and prevent falls. Tai chi (page 38) has been shown to lower the risk of falls.

Be aware that those who drink alcohol are at a higher risk of injuries and falls. If you do find that you have osteoporosis and feel unsteady, consider wearing hip protectors (see page 131). Hip protectors are simple underwear that has been shown to lower the risk of hip fracture by 50 percent if you happen to fall.

Prevention strategy 5: Use an integrative medicine approach. Taking advantage of the most effective conventional medicine and safe, natural therapies can give you the best bone-building benefit. Review your need for natural dietary supplements, making sure you get 1,000 mg of calcium if you are age twenty-five to sixty-five, and 1,500 mg if you are over sixty-five. Also get 400 IU of vitamin D in your daily diet. If you are taking medications such as prednisone, consider one of the bone-strengthening medications in Step 5. Medications that treat osteoporosis in women have also been shown to be effective in bone building for men, which can help to lower your risk of painful and debilitating fractures.

Osteoporosis does not just affect women. Men get painful fractures, lose height, and, more important, lose independence and quality of life. Take action! Talk with your doctor and take steps to prevent osteoporosis and fractures so you can live an active and independent life—the rest of your life.

Special Situation 4: Spinal Fractures and Back Pain

Back pain is nothing new to most Americans. It's estimated that back pain affects four out of five adults at some point in their lifetime. As we discuss in our *The Pain-Free Back* (Owl), back pain is the most common reason people visit their doctors. In the United States, back pain is:

- The most prevalent cause of disability in men and women under age 45
- The nation's number one occupational hazard
- The third most frequent reason for surgical procedures
- The reason for more lost work days than any other ailment except arthritis and related diseases

A common cause of acute back pain is a spinal fracture resulting from osteoporosis. As discussed previously, spinal fractures can be painful. Not only do they cause loss of height, a stooped posture, and dowager's hump (see page 9), they add to your medical cost and even increase your risk of other medical problems.

By age seventy-five, 50 percent or more of all women have had a fracture in their spine, most commonly from osteoporosis. Ironically, most of these spinal fractures are silent and do not cause pain. However, when they do cause pain, it is severe and usually strikes suddenly. The fracture may happen after lifting, such as opening a window, or after a fall. However, the pain that follows may be so severe that walking, sitting, and standing are almost impossible. This pain can be incapacitating for days or even weeks until the fracture heals. We find that many patients who suffer with spinal fractures and back pain have difficulty sleeping and sometimes require pain medication for relief.

The pain of the spinal fracture may feel worse when you cough or sneeze but does not usually travel down one leg (sciatica). Let your doctor know if you have this feeling, as it may be a sign of pressure on a nerve.

Chronic back pain can lead to problems with simply bending over, lifting a child or bag of groceries, walking up or down stairs, or even just standing at the kitchen counter. Fear of falling can loom large after spine fracture.

Finding Relief

Relief of pain is usually best if you stay in a reclining position instead of lying flat or sitting up—you want to be about halfway in between. Find the most comfortable position and in a few days the pain will lessen. Usually within a few weeks, the pain will be manageable without narcotics. If not, check with your doctor to see if some other treatment might be needed.

Exercise and Diet Speed Recovery

As soon as the pain allows, you can begin to move around, walking through your home, gradually increasing the time you spend on your feet, and eventually embracing other activities. It's now time to take steps toward preventing additional fractures by starting your Bone-Building Workout (Step 2). Go very slowly at first to avoid further injury.

Make sure your diet has the proper amount of calcium and vitamin D and add a medication, as discussed in Step 5, if necessary to increase bone strength and lower fracture risk. Some medications are effective in lowering the risk of spine fractures by 65 to 70 percent within one year.

More Than One Fracture

As more information about the risk of spine fractures becomes available, it's clear that our ultimate goal should be to prevent the first fracture altogether. We know that having one spine fracture greatly increases your risk of having another—and another. Researchers have shown that about one in five people who have one spine fracture may have another one within twelve months. Studies also show that the spine fracture will increase the chance of other fractures, including hip fractures.

Even though treatment is available for all of these conditions and even though it is never too late to prevent the next fracture, the best-case scenario is to stop osteoporosis before it happens. This can be done if you find low bone mass early from your bone density test and begin treatment for osteopenia. Considering the consequences, it is no wonder that so many women and men now want to be proactive in their treatment of low bone mass and osteopenia.

What You Might Feel

If you have more than one spinal fracture, your pain may be more severe. The fracture may affect more than one area of the spine, or it can last longer than a few weeks. When more than one fracture happens from osteoporosis and no other causes are found, then medications can be started to control pain and prevent future fractures. Treatments such as vertebroplasty and kyphoplasty are also available (page 143).

Other Signs and Symptoms

After several spine fractures, loss of height can lead to the classic dowager's hump. In fact, with each spine fracture, you can lose an average of one-quarter inch of your height. After enough height loss, the stomach may be compressed and protrude out over the rib cage. This can be quite uncomfortable, causing poor appetite, shortness of breath, and difficulty fitting into the clothes you've worn for years.

Get an Accurate Diagnosis

Even if you have osteoporosis, your back pain may stem from a different source. Acute back pain commonly stems from problems with the muscles, tendons, and ligaments around the back—the soft tissues, not the bones of the spine. These and other causes of back pain can happen with or without a fracture in the spine. Your doctor can help you sort out the problem.

It's very common to have more than one cause of back pain. For example, you might have back pain from a spine fracture and osteoarthritis (the "wear and tear" arthritis). Or you could have back pain from a spine fracture and a muscle injury from years ago. Other less common causes of back pain include infection or cancer. It is important to discuss the possible causes with your doctor.

It's essential to get an accurate diagnosis, because there are good treatments available—different treatments for different causes of back pain.

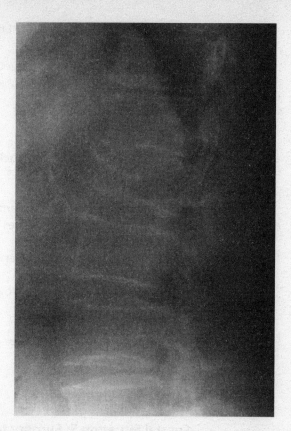

Figure 6.1

X ray of a fracture of a lumbar vertebra

There are tests available to help diagnose the causes of back pain beyond examination by your doctor.

X rays. When you have back pain, X rays are the quickest and easiest way to find a spine fracture. X rays will show one of the bones of the spine to be shortened with a different shape (see X ray above). You can see why these fractures can lead to shortening of the spine and loss of height.

Magnetic resonance imaging (MRI). Magnetic resonance imaging (MRI) is another diagnostic test that can show more accurate details of the bones of the spine than an X ray. An MRI can reveal problems such as infection, cancer, pressure on a nerve, or other medical problems causing back pain and may also give an idea whether the fracture is acute or not.

Computerized tomography (CT) scan. The CT scan provides a detailed picture of the spine fracture and can help eliminate possible causes of a fracture or back pain.

Other laboratory tests. Your doctor may ask for other laboratory tests, such as blood and urine tests, to see if there are any other medical problems causing fractures in the spine.

Be sure you talk with your doctor and give feedback if your pain doesn't improve or you cannot resume your normal activities. Find the other problems and begin treatment to target what's causing your back pain. Using the most effective treatment for each cause can bring the best and most complete relief of your pain.

Common Causes of Back Pain

Fracture from osteoporosis
Problems with muscles, tendons, and ligaments around the back
Problems with trigger areas in the soft tissues around the back
Osteoarthritis in the spine
True sciatica-ruptured disk (pressure on a nerve in the lower spine that radiates into a leg)
Lumbar stenosis (pressure on nerves in the lower back from narrowing of the spine)
Fibromyalgia
Other types of arthritis
Other medical problems

Special Situation 5: Surgery for Fractures

If your doctor recommends surgery, it's important to understand all you can about the invasive procedure. The goals of surgery in an osteoporotic fracture include:

- Pain relief
- Physical rehabilitation and return to your prior level of activity
- Preventing a second fracture

Your doctor will refer you to a surgeon if you have a fracture, such as a broken hip after a fall onto a weak, osteoporotic bone. You might also see a surgeon for evaluation if pain persists despite attempts to treat with medication. An imaging study, such as an X ray or even a CT scan or MRI, may shed light on the true source of the pain.

Surgical Management of Vertebral Fractures

Thirty percent of patients with spinal fractures will notice an immediate, sharp pain in the area of the back with the broken vertebrae. This acute pain usually lasts a few weeks, but may last up to twelve weeks. Chronic pain can be caused by muscle spasm around the area of fracture, arthritis that develops around a broken vertebra, or changes in overall spinal alignment. With progressive loss of height, your center of gravity may shift, which can affect the way you walk and necessitate at least temporary use of a cane or walker.

Exercise programs have been shown to decrease the need for pain medicine, improve quality of life, and even increase bone density. A walking regimen or the ancient discipline of tai chi may be beneficial after the pain is controlled. If pain cannot be controlled adequately by oral medications, hospitalization may be necessary to provide intravenous pain relief.

In years past, when medications failed there were no other options for those suffering from one or several disabling spine fractures. Recently two procedures called vertebroplasty and kyphoplasty have arisen to treat an acute (new) or painful vertebral fracture associated with osteoporosis. The development of these two minimally invasive procedures has evoked both excitement and controversy.

The goal of both techniques is to relieve the acute pain of a spine fracture, if it doesn't improve after a few weeks. Pain relief is good in about 80 to 90 percent of patients. There also has not yet been proven long-term benefit, when compared to simple, traditional treatment for a spine fracture.

Vertebroplasty

Vertebroplasty involves directly injecting a certain kind of bone cement, called polymethylmethacrylate (PMMA), into the fractured area of the vertebral body. This procedure is most commonly performed by an interventional radiologist under guidance of fluoroscopy, a specific kind of X-ray imaging. The acrylic cement is injected under a high pressure into the partially collapsed vertebral body. Vertebroplasty may reduce pain in the immediate period after the procedure, usually with a difference in pain relief noted in the first twenty-four hours.

With vertebroplasty, there is no restoration of loss of height. Multiple spine fractures can be treated at one session. Considered a relatively simple procedure, vertebroplasty is often done under local anesthesia. In other words, you can carry on a conversation with the physician during the procedure.

Most patients experience no problems, but the most common complication of vertebroplasty is leakage of cement into nearby nerves. Greater cement leakage occurs with vertebroplasty than lower-pressure kyphoplasty. Short-term problems could include more pain, or damage to a nearby nerve or the spinal cord due to heat or pressure from the needle. Long-term complications are not clear, but may include a possible increased risk of fracture in vertebrae adjacent to the one treated. In either case, you must be able to tolerate lying prone on the stomach for a couple of hours. General anesthesia is used if lying prone is a problem. For simple treatment, intravenous sedation and local anesthesia are usually adequate.

Kyphoplasty

Kyphoplasty, a newer technique, was developed from vertebroplasty. The goals of kyphoplasty are to relieve pain and to reexpand the vertebral body to regain height. Instead of using a long needle to inject the cement into the vertebra, with kyphoplasty an inflatable balloonlike catheter is inserted into the vertebra to expand the previously collapsed body before injecting the bone cement.

An orthopedic surgeon usually performs kyphoplasty. Again, pain relief is experienced in about 80 to 90 percent of patients, with 70 percent regaining lost vertebral height.

Long-Term Forecast

We await longer trials of these two procedures. Until better understood, we feel that vertebroplasty and kyphoplasty are best reserved for carefully selected patients and done only by an experienced specialist. Optimally, a patient would have a persistent, deep, intense pain over a few weeks at the area of the spinal fracture noted on an X ray or MRI. While they both offer immediate pain relief, there are no studies showing that long-term pain control or physical function is better with these procedures.

Surgical Management of Hip Fracture

Timely surgery is paramount in managing hip fractures because the goals of early intervention and rapid physical rehabilitation allow the best chance to restore prior level of function. If surgery is an option after a fall with a hip fracture, then the best timing is usually within the first 48 hours after the injury. Prior to the surgery, your physician will evaluate you for other active medical problems such as diabetes, high blood pressure, or heart disease.

The current trend after hip surgery is avoiding prolonged immobilization. Trained therapists work with patients soon after the procedure.

After hip fracture, the most common procedure involves internal fixation with hardware (rods and screws) placed into the bone to give it strong support. In most cases, operating on a broken hip with internal fixation usually has better results than no surgery at all. However, this decision should be made by the orthopedic surgeon. Sometimes bone grafting is also done with this surgery. With bone grafting, bone is taken from another bone (usually the iliac crest, which is part of the pelvis in the low back or hip area). This bone graft can stimulate new bone to grow at the site of the fracture, subsequently reducing the risk of another fracture. Bone cement is used with the hardware to ensure long-term support at the site of the fracture.

Sometimes a hip fracture in a younger, more physically active person can be treated with an operation involving a total hip replacement (THR). In this case, a prosthetic hip joint replaces the broken hip. The results are usually remarkable, with good pain relief and range of motion.

Pre-Op Screening

Before surgery, you will probably undergo pre-op screening tests, which may include the following:

1. Basic blood work, including blood counts, kidney function, and blood glucose
2. Electrocardiogram (EKG)
3. Chest X ray
4. Urine analysis
5. Pregnancy test (if premenopausal female)

Other tests will be determined by your doctor, depending on any coexisting medical problems, medications, your age, and the type and urgency of the surgery.

Surgical Management of Shoulder Fracture

The upper part of the arm (near the shoulder), or humerus, is another bone more likely to break when the bone density is low. Compared to a hip fracture, a broken humerus usually heals well without surgery. In fact,

about 80 percent of patients heal with just a brief period of immobilization (that is, the patient wears a shoulder sling).

If the humeral fracture is severe, surgery might be considered. Aggres-
sive physical rehabilitation is paramount in either case to avoid a stiff,
frozen shoulder. If range of motion is not returned, you can lose the ability
to perform daily tasks of life, including dressing yourself.

Postoperative Care

Sometimes it's impractical to return home after surgery, particularly after
a hip fracture or if your pre-injury level of function was already limited.
Short-term physical therapy (up to a few weeks) at a rehabilitation center
may be helpful.

In general, bearing weight or walking after surgery is limited only for a
short time. Using a walker with careful instruction and assistance of a trained
therapist can give you more independence and an increased range of motion.
The therapist will also discuss proper body mechanics and alert you to specific activities to avoid including bending, lifting, and pushing.

Meet the Anesthesiologist

It is standard to meet with the anesthesiologist prior to surgery, usually
during the preoperative exam. This professional monitors your breathing and blood pressure among other things during the surgery. Be sure
to communicate the following with this doctor:

- Health problems you may have (lung disease, heart problems, chronic
  illness)
- Previous problems with anesthesia
- If you desire to be awake during surgery

Managing Pain after Surgery

After surgery, the goal is early return to at least low-impact activity as
directed specifically by the surgeon and physical therapist. He or she will
prescribe additional physical therapy and exercises that are crucial to
resuming your daily activities as quickly as possible. Be sure to ask your
doctor when you can return to specific activities, such as your exercise

regimen or duties at work. If you are caring for children, make sure you have help available until your doctor allows you to safely lift again.

In addition to local healing of any surgical incision, the goal should include "preventive maintenance." The ideal way to approach recovery from any surgery, in addition to adequate analgesia with medications prescribed by the surgeon or your physician, include:

1. *Treat the cause of the pain.* For example, you have to treat the osteoporosis to prevent another fracture. Educating yourself on what osteoporosis is, and then seeing your doctor for a bone mineral density (BMD) test, if you are at risk, are both important prevention measures. If your BMD is too low, make sure you get ample calcium and vitamin D, following the guidelines in Step 3. Newer medications can decrease the chance of having another bone fracture by over 50 percent. Contrary to what you might think, bed rest can actually lead to loss of bone mineral density, so slowly but gradually increase activity to prevent worsening osteoporosis.

2. *Decrease risk of falling.* You would hate to undergo successful surgery, and then slip and fall at home while walking from the mailbox to the front door. Review the suggestions for fall-proofing your home and make sure your living environment won't add to your pain.

3. *Continue the exercises recommended in your Bone-Building Workout (Step 2).* Low-impact exercises even after surgery, if directed by a physical therapist, may speed post-op recovery. Aquatics or water exercises are an ideal way to increase aerobic capacity and strength after surgery with minimal force to the healing body.

4. *Lose excess weight.* Being at a normal weight is most helpful before surgery to decrease surgical complications. It helps after surgery as well, to decrease the heavy load on your recovering body.

CHAPTER 7

Bone-Building Recipes

No matter how healthy—or unhealthy—your current diet is, we want to show you some creative and easy ways to make tasty changes that give you variety and the right nutrients proven to keep bones strong. Whether you are a vegetarian or a meat eater who wants to reduce (not eliminate) the amount of meat in your diet, the following Bone-Building Recipes will start you and your family on the right track to staying strong your entire lifetime.

Drinks/Appetizers
Sweet Mango Drink
Peanut Butter and Jelly Shake

Breads
Strawberry Muffins
Savory Harvest Muffins
Zucchini Nut Muffins
Bruschetta with a Twist

Soups
Seafood Chowder
Asian Vegetable Soup
Black and White Soup
Creamy Tomato Soup

Salads/Sauces
Egg Salad on Spinach
Spicy Chicken Salad
Greek Salad
Easy Antipasto
Colorful Pasta Salad
Peanut Sauce

Pasta/Rice
Eggplant Parmesan with Angel
    Hair Pasta
Penne with Glorious Greens
Fettuccine Alfredo
Indian Dal
Tofu Noodles with Peanut Sauce
Tabouleh

Entrees

Grilled Salmon with Fresh Herbs
Asian Grilled Tuna Burgers
Surprise Pesto Chicken
    Sandwiches
Mediterranean Chicken with
    Spinach and Feta
Creamed Chicken Tortilla Bake
Zesty Quesadillas
Pastitsio
Beef Stroganoff
Baked Spaghetti
Sweet and Sour Meatballs
Eggs Benedict
Vegetarian Sausage and Pepperoni
    Pizza

Vegetables

Asparagus with Lemon and
    Parmesan

Creamy Artichoke Dip
Summer Squash Gratin
Colorful Roasted Peppers
Roasted Parsnips
Rice and Peas
Indian Curried Sweet Potato
Spinach and Corn Pastry
Hearty Vegetable Walnut Spread
Mom's Baked Beans
Mother Mac's Elegant Carrots
Broccoli Quiche

Desserts

Fried Bananas
Sweet Strawberry Pie
Peanut Butter Cookies
Fruit and Nut Cake

DRINKS/APPETIZERS

✤ Sweet Mango Drink

Ingredients
1 cup pineapple juice
1 ripe mango
Lime and sugar to taste

Directions
Place ingredients in blender and liquefy. Serve immediately.

Yield: Serves 2.

Nutritional information per serving: Calories: 124, Fat: <1g,
    Carbohydrates: 31g, Fiber: 2g, Protein: 1g.

❖ Peanut Butter and Jelly Shake

Ingredients
2 cups low-fat milk
2 tablespoons peanut butter
1½ cups frozen strawberries
2 bananas
1 tablespoon flaxseeds

Directions
Place all ingredients in a blender and blend until thick and creamy. Serve immediately.

Yield: Serves 3.

Nutritional information per serving: Calories: 257, Fat: 7g, Carbohydrates: 33g, Fiber: 4g, Protein: 11g.

BREADS

❖ Strawberry Muffins

Ingredients
1½ cups white pastry flour
½ cup wheat flour
3 teaspoons baking powder
½ cup white sugar
1 cup low-fat milk
3 tablespoons canola oil
1 egg, beaten
1 cup chopped strawberries, drizzled with honey

Directions
Preheat oven to 375 degrees. Combine dry ingredients in a large mixing bowl. Stir to combine. Pour milk, oil, and egg into a small bowl and stir. Combine all ingredients and stir well with a fork. Fill paper muffin cups ⅔ full with batter. Bake for 25–30 minutes, until cooked through.

Yield: 12 muffins.

Nutritional information per serving: Calories: 166, Fat: 4g, Carbohydrates: 29g, Fiber: 1g, Protein: 3g.

❖ Harvest Muffins

Ingredients
2 cups white pastry flour, sifted
3 teaspoons baking powder
½ teaspoon salt
½ cup canned pumpkin
½ cup sugar
1 egg
½ cup low-fat milk
¼ cup canola oil
½ teaspoon fresh ground nutmeg
1 teaspoon fresh ground cinnamon

FILLING:
4 ounces Neufchatel cheese
1 tablespoon low-fat milk
1 tablespoon sugar

Directions
Preheat oven to 375 degrees. Place flour, baking powder, and salt in a small mixing bowl. Stir to combine. In a large bowl, blend pumpkin, sugar, egg, milk, and oil. Add dry ingredients to bowl and stir again. Stir in nutmeg and cinnamon. Pour batter into muffin cups, and fill ⅔ full.

For filling, combine Neufchatel cheese, milk, and sugar and mix well. Place 1 tablespoon of filling in the middle of each muffin cup. Use knife to make a swirl pattern in each muffin. Bake muffins 25–30 minutes until cooked through.

Yield: 12 muffins.

Nutritional information per serving: Calories: 183, Fat: 7g, Carbohydrates: 27g, Fiber: <1g, Protein: 4g.

❖ Zucchini Nut Muffins

Ingredients
1⅓ cups zucchini, chopped
1½ cups flour
½ teaspoon baking soda
½ teaspoon salt
2 eggs
⅓ cup canola oil
½ banana, chopped
¼ cup apple juice
⅔ cup white sugar
½ teaspoon cinnamon
½ cup pecans, chopped
½ cup raisins

Directions
In a food processor, grate zucchini until it is chopped very fine. Combine flour, baking soda, and salt in a small bowl. In a large mixing bowl, blend eggs, oil, banana, apple juice, sugar, and cinnamon. Add dry ingredients to the large mixing bowl and stir with a spoon. Pour in pecans and raisins and stir again. Fill muffin cups ⅔ full and bake for 25 minutes at 375 degrees, until inserted toothpick comes out clean. Serve with butter or nut butter.

Yield: 12 muffins.

Nutritional information per serving: Calories: 219, Fat: 9g, Carbohydrates: 33g, Fiber: 1g, Protein: 3g.

❖ Bruschetta with a Twist

Ingredients
1 cup Roma tomatoes, deseeded, diced
2 garlic cloves, minced
2 tablespoons olive oil
1 large baguette, cut in 12 thick slices
¼ cup fresh basil, chopped

Salt and pepper to taste
Optional garnishes: pine nuts, olives, feta, capers, or thick slices of buffalo
   mozzarella

Directions
Mix tomatoes, garlic, olive oil, and salt and pepper in a small bowl.
Marinate for several hours. Before serving, toast baguette slices lightly and
place on a serving plate. Spoon tomato mixture onto bread and sprinkle
with fresh basil. Add toppings if desired.

Yield: Serves 6.

Nutritional information per serving: Calories: 187, Fat: 6g, Carbohydrates:
   26g, Fiber: 2g, Protein: 5g.

SOUPS

✤ Seafood Chowder

Ingredients
1 tablespoon canola oil
1 large white onion, diced
2 large celery stalks, sliced thinly
2 cloves garlic, minced
2 cups vegetable broth
2 cups potatoes, peeled and chopped in small cubes
2 large carrots, peeled and sliced thinly
2 tablespoons fresh dill, chopped finely
2 cups cooked fresh salmon, bones removed (or 16 ounces canned
   salmon, drained)
1 15-ounce can creamed corn
1 12-ounce can evaporated skim milk
¾ cup cheddar cheese, shredded
Salt and pepper to taste

Directions
In a large pot heat oil, onion, celery, and garlic on medium heat. Sauté 3–5
minutes until onion turns golden. Add vegetable broth, potatoes, carrots,

and dill. Heat to a boil then reduce heat to a simmer. Cover and cook for 25 minutes. Add salmon, corn, milk, and cheese and cook, covered, for 10 minutes until heated through. Add salt and pepper to taste.

Yield: Serves 8.

Nutritional information per serving: Calories: 278, Fat: 11g, Carbohydrates: 30g, Fiber: 3g, Protein: 18g.

❖ Asian Vegetable Soup

Ingredients
2 tablespoons sesame oil
1 16-ounce package firm tofu, drained, chopped in small cubes
2 tablespoons soy sauce
1 tablespoon garlic powder
1 tablespoon sesame oil
½ cup yellow onion, sliced
1 cup carrots, sliced thinly
½ tablespoon fresh ginger, minced
2 cloves garlic, minced
3 cups vegetable broth
½–1 teaspoon crushed red pepper flakes
2 cups fresh spinach, washed, chopped
1 cup bean sprouts
½ cup crushed peanuts

Directions
Pour 2 tablespoons of the sesame oil into a large wok or saucepan. Heat on medium high and add tofu, stir-frying for 5–10 minutes until tofu turns golden brown, flipping once. Turn off heat and stir in soy sauce and garlic powder. Lay tofu in a single layer on paper towels to drain. In a large saucepan, combine 1 tablespoon sesame oil, onion, carrots, ginger, and garlic and cook on medium heat. Stir-fry vegetables until onion turns translucent, 3–5 minutes. Pour vegetable stock into the pot. Stir in tofu and crushed red pepper. Heat to boiling, then turn heat down to a simmer for 10 minutes. Stir in spinach. Add more soy sauce and/or water to taste. Garnish with bean sprouts and crushed peanuts.

Yield: Serves 4.

Nutritional information per serving: Calories: 342, Fat: 27g,
   Carbohydrates: 11g, Fiber: 5g, Protein: 18g.

✤ Yin and Yang Soup

Ingredients
2 15-ounce cans black beans, drained
2 cups vegetable broth
1 white onion, diced
1 green pepper, diced
1 cup fresh salsa
1 teaspoon onion powder
1 tablespoon garlic powder
1 teaspoon sugar
Juice of one lime
1 cup whole milk
1 pound Mexican melting cheese, cubed (or substitute Velveeta)
2–3 tablespoons fresh jalapenos, minced (optional)
Salt and hot sauce to taste

Directions
Combine black beans, vegetable broth, onion, green pepper, and salsa in a
large pot. Bring to a boil, then cover, simmering for 15 minutes. Add onion
powder, garlic powder, sugar, and lime juice. Stir well and let sit for several
minutes while preparing the white soup. In a smaller pot on medium low
heat, cook milk and cheese for 5–7 minutes, stirring occasionally. Season
with salt and hot sauce as desired. Stir in jalapenos. Transfer black bean
soup to a blender and pulse until soup is mostly creamy. To serve, scoop
black bean soup and white soup with separate ladles, and then pour side by
side into a serving bowl. Top with salsa, sour cream, and cilantro.

Yield: Serves 8.

Nutritional information per serving: Calories: 342, Fat: 17g,
   Carbohydrates: 28g, Fiber: 9g, Protein: 22g.

❖ Creamy Tomato Soup

Ingredients
1 tablespoon olive oil
1 small onion, diced
3 cloves garlic, minced
1 tablespoon flour
28 ounces canned plum tomatoes, with liquid
1½ cups vegetable stock
3 tablespoons tomato paste
1 tablespoon sugar
¼ cup fresh basil, chopped
1 tablespoon garlic powder
1 tablespoon onion powder
1 cup half-and-half
Salt and pepper to taste

Directions
Heat olive oil in a large pot on medium heat. Add onion and garlic and stir, cooking until onion is translucent. Stir in flour and cook for 1 minute. Stir in plum tomatoes with liquid, vegetable stock, tomato paste, and sugar. Stir to combine and bring to a boil. Add basil and seasonings and allow to simmer on medium-low heat for 25 minutes, stirring occasionally. Turn off heat and allow to cool slightly. Pour soup into blender in separate batches and pulse until smooth. Return soup to pot and add half-and-half. Stir well and simmer until heated through.

Yield: Serves 5.

Nutritional information per serving: Calories: 170, Fat: 9g, Carbohydrates: 21g, Fiber: 3g, Protein: 4g.

SALADS/SAUCES

❖ Egg Salad on Spinach

Ingredients
6 hard-boiled eggs, peeled
3 tablespoons mayonnaise

1 tablespoon yellow mustard
2 tablespoons relish
¼ cup celery, sliced thinly
¼ cup green olives, sliced thinly
3 cups fresh spinach, washed and torn into bite-size pieces
Salt and pepper to taste

Directions
Mash eggs in a mixing bowl with mayonnaise, mustard, and relish. Stir in celery and olives. Add salt and pepper to taste. Serve on beds of fresh spinach or on toast.

Yield: Serves 3.

Nutritional information per serving: Calories: 226, Fat: 16g, Carbohydrates: 7g, Fiber: 2g, Protein: 14g.

❖ Spicy Chicken Salad

Ingredients
1 head green-leaf lettuce, chopped in small pieces
2 cups shredded cooked chicken
1 cup chopped fresh tomato
½ cup green onions, chopped
¼ cup Monterey Jack with pepper cheese, shredded
¼ cup sharp cheddar cheese, shredded
¼ cup chopped fresh cilantro
1 avocado, pitted, sliced
Jalapenos for garnish, if desired

Directions
Layer lettuce in a large salad bowl. Top with chicken, tomato, green onions, and cheese. Sprinkle cilantro on top and garnish with avocado and jalapeno peppers. Serve with a creamy southwestern dressing.

Yield: Serves 4.

Nutritional information per serving: Calories: 321, Fat: 20g, Carbohydrates: 9g, Fiber: 5g, Protein: 29g.

❖ Greek Salad

Ingredients
1 large head romaine lettuce
½ cup cucumber, chopped
¼ cup green pepper, chopped
¼ cup red onion, sliced
½ cup olives, green or black, sliced
1 large tomato, sliced
1 cup feta cheese, crumbled

Directions
Tear lettuce into bite-sized pieces. Toss with vegetables in a large serving bowl. Top with feta cheese and serve with your favorite Italian dressing.

Yield: Serves 6.

Nutritional information per serving: Calories: 94, Fat: 2g, Carbohydrates: 4g, Fiber: 2g, Protein: 2g.

❖ Easy Antipasto

Ingredients
1 16-ounce jar roasted red peppers, drained, sliced
½ cup sun-dried tomatoes, reconstituted, drained, diced
1 7-ounce jar artichoke hearts, drained, quartered
1 7-ounce jar mushrooms, drained
1 cup olives (any variety)
4 ounces turkey or soy pepperoni slices
8 ounces boneless, lean ham, sliced thin
1 cup fresh buffalo mozzarella, sliced
½ cup Parmesan, sliced

DRESSING:
¼ cup red wine vinegar
⅓ cup olive oil
2 tablespoons fresh basil, chopped

1 tablespoon fresh rosemary, chopped
1 clove garlic, minced
½–1 teaspoon crushed red pepper
1 tablespoon lemon juice
1 teaspoon salt
1 teaspoon sugar

Directions
Arrange all vegetables, meats, and cheeses on a large platter. Combine dressing ingredients and mix well. Spoon dressing over antipasto as desired.

Yield: Serves 8.

Nutritional information per serving: Calories: 249, Fat: 16g, Carbohydrates: 10g, Fiber: 3g, Protein: 17g.

❖ Colorful Pasta Salad

Ingredients
12 ounces cheese tortellini, any variety
2 tablespoons olive oil
2 cloves garlic, minced
½ cup shredded carrots
¼ cup yellow squash, chopped finely
¼ cup asparagus tips, chopped finely
¼ cup red pepper, chopped finely
½ cup fresh or canned corn

DRESSING:
3 tablespoons sun-dried tomato tapenade
2 tablespoons white wine vinegar
3 tablespoons olive oil
1 tablespoon fresh lemon juice
1 teaspoon dried rosemary
1 teaspoon onion powder
Salt and pepper to taste

Directions
Heat water in a large pot and cook tortellini according to package directions, then drain. Drizzle with 1 tablespoon olive oil, toss gently, and set aside. In a small saucepan, stir in 1 tablespoon olive oil, garlic, carrots, squash, asparagus, red pepper, and corn. Cook on medium heat 5–7 minutes, until vegetables are crisp-tender. In a large mixing bowl, stir pasta, vegetables, and dressing ingredients together. Mix well. Refrigerate for several hours or overnight.

Yield: Serves 6.

Nutritional information per serving: Calories: 296, Fat: 14g, Carbohydrates: 33g, Fiber: 4g, Protein: 6g.

❖ Peanut Sauce

Ingredients
½ tablespoon canola oil
½ cup yellow onion, diced
2 garlic cloves, minced
¼ cup creamy peanut butter
½ cup coconut milk
½ tablespoon white sugar
1 tablespoon rice vinegar
1 tablespoon soy sauce
1 teaspoon lemongrass, chopped
½–1 teaspoon red pepper

Directions
Heat oil in a large saucepan and add onion and garlic. Stir-fry for several minutes until onions are golden and translucent. Add peanut butter, coconut milk, sugar, vinegar, soy sauce, and spices and stir well. Cook on medium-low heat for 5 minutes until smooth and creamy, stirring occasionally. Mix in blender for a smoother sauce. Serve with pasta or vegetables.

Yield: Serves 4.

Nutritional information per serving: Calories: 175, Fat: 17g,
Carbohydrates: 7g, Fiber: 1g, Protein: 5g.

PASTA/RICE

❖ Eggplant Parmesan with Angel Hair Pasta

Ingredients
1 medium-size eggplant
2 tablespoons olive oil
1 large onion, diced
1 red pepper, diced
4 cloves garlic, minced
1 teaspoon oregano
1 26-ounce can tomato sauce
2 large ripe tomatoes, deseeded, chopped
¼ cup grated Parmesan cheese
8 ounces mozzarella cheese, shredded
12 ounces angel hair pasta
Salt and pepper to taste

Directions
Wash and cut eggplant in thin slices. Spread evenly on a flat pan. Sprinkle
salt over eggplant, then flip over and sprinkle with salt again. Cover with a
layer of paper towels. Place a large pan over the eggplant and place heavy
items on top of the pan so the eggplant slices are pressed down flat. Allow
to sit for at least 1 hour.

In a large pan, heat 1 tablespoon olive oil and toss in onions. Cook until
onion turns translucent. Stir in red pepper and garlic. Cook for several
minutes, then add oregano, tomato sauce, and tomatoes. Add salt and
pepper to taste. Stir well and cook, covered, for 20–30 minutes until
sauce thickens.

While sauce is cooking, heat 1 tablespoon olive oil in a large pan. Place
eggplant slices in pan and cook until golden brown, turning once to cook
both sides. Repeat until all eggplant slices are cooked. Drain on paper
towels.

Spoon ⅓ of the tomato sauce into a large baking dish. Cover with half of the eggplant slices and sprinkle with Parmesan cheese. Spoon ⅓ of the tomato sauce on the cheese and layer with the other eggplant slices. Cover with remaining sauce and sprinkle mozzarella cheese on top. Cover with foil and bake at 375 degrees for 30–40 minutes. While eggplant is baking, cook pasta according to package directions. Remove foil from eggplant and cook for 10–15 minutes or until moisture is absorbed and cheese is lightly browned. Serve over angel hair pasta.

Yield: Serves 6.

Nutritional information per serving: Calories: 456, Fat: 15g, Carbohydrates: 62g, Fiber: 11g, Protein: 21g.

❖ Penne Pasta with Stir-Fry Greens

Ingredients
8 ounces penne pasta
2 tablespoons olive oil
1 red onion, chopped
1 red pepper, chopped
3 cloves garlic, minced
4 cups green leafy vegetables (kale, spinach, and/or chard)
1 tablespoon fresh thyme, chopped
½ cup Parmesan cheese, freshly grated
Salt and pepper to taste

Directions
Cook pasta according to package directions. Heat oil in a large pot and sauté onion, red pepper, and garlic for several minutes, until onion and red pepper begin to soften. Stir in greens and thyme. Stir well and cover, cooking for several minutes until the greens begin to wilt slightly. Toss pasta with vegetables in a large serving bowl. Season with salt and pepper and sprinkle with Parmesan cheese.

Yield: Serves 4.

Nutritional information per serving: Calories: 317, Fat: 11g, Carbohydrates: 49g, Fiber: 7g, Protein: 10g.

❖ Fettuccine Alfredo

Ingredients
8 ounces fettuccine pasta
3 tablespoons butter or margarine
¼ cup white flour
2 cups low-fat milk
¼ cup shredded mozzarella cheese
½ cup grated Parmesan cheese
1 cup broccoli florets, chopped, steamed
Salt and pepper to taste

Directions
Prepare pasta according to package directions. Melt butter in a small saucepan on medium heat. Add flour and stir constantly for 1 minute or until light gold in color. In a separate pan, warm milk on low heat, then pour milk into the flour-butter mixture. Stir well until lumps of flour dissolve. Add cheeses. Cook on medium heat and stir often as sauce thickens, 3–4 minutes. Reduce heat to low and add salt and pepper to taste. Cook on low heat for several minutes more, stirring occasionally. Toss pasta with sauce and steamed broccoli.

Yield: Serves 4.

Nutritional information per serving: Calories: 439, Fat: 14g, Carbohydrates: 55g, Fiber: 6g, Protein: 19g.

❖ Lentil Dal

Ingredients
1 tablespoon canola oil
1 white onion, finely diced
1 teaspoon ground cinnamon
1 teaspoon ground cumin
1 cup yellow lentils
3 cups water
1 cup plain yogurt
3 cups cooked brown rice

1 tablespoon fresh cilantro, chopped
Salt to taste

Directions
Add oil, onion, cinnamon, and cumin to a large pot and cook on medium heat for 2 minutes. Add lentils and water and bring to a boil. Cover and simmer for 1–2 hours until lentils are smooth and creamy. Serve over rice and spoon plain yogurt on top. Sprinkle with cilantro.

Yield: Serves 6.

Nutritional information per serving: Calories: 279, Fat: 4g, Carbohydrates: 49g, Fiber: 6g, Protein: 12g.

❖ Tofu Peanut Noodles

Ingredients
1 tablespoon sesame oil
1 16-ounce block firm tofu, drained, cut in ½-inch thick slices
1 tablespoon sesame oil
1 small yellow onion, diced
1 carrot, grated
1 red pepper, diced
1 cup broccoli florets, chopped
2 cups spinach, washed, drained, chopped
1 batch Peanut Sauce, see page 160
8 ounces rice noodles
Soy sauce, to taste
Crushed red pepper, to taste
3 tablespoons crushed peanuts
⅓ cup bean sprouts, washed

Directions
Heat 1 tablespoon sesame oil in a large pan. Add tofu slices and cook for several minutes on each side until crispy and golden brown. Drain on paper towels. Heat 1 tablespoon sesame oil in a large pan and add onion and carrots. Cook for several minutes until vegetables begin to soften. Add red pepper and broccoli and stir well. Sauté for several minutes. Add

spinach to pot and cover, cooking until spinach is wilted. Stir, turn off heat, and set aside. Cook rice noodles according to package directions. Toss cooked noodles with vegetables and prepared peanut sauce. Season with soy sauce and crushed red pepper as desired. Garnish with peanuts and sprouts.

Yield: Serves 5.

Nutritional information per serving: Calories: 359, Fat: 12g, Carbohydrates: 45g, Fiber: 5g, Protein: 15g.

✤ Tabouleh

Ingredients
1 cup bulgur wheat
2 cups boiling water
2–3 green onions, diced
2 large tomatoes, deseeded, chopped
1 medium cucumber, chopped
1 cup fresh parsley, finely chopped
¼ cup fresh mint, finely chopped
¼ cup fresh lemon juice
2 tablespoons olive oil
Salt and pepper to taste

Directions
Place bulgur wheat in a large mixing bowl and cover with 2 cups boiling water. Let sit for at least 30 minutes, until water is absorbed. Fluff with a fork. Add all other ingredients and mix well. Refrigerate for several hours or overnight.

Yield: Serves 8.

Nutritional information per serving: Calories: 113, Fat: 3g, Carbohydrates: 19g, Fiber: 5g, Protein: 3g.

ENTREES

❖ Grilled Salmon with Fresh Herbs

Ingredients
1 pound salmon fillets
2 tablespoons fresh cilantro
2 tablespoons fresh parsley
2 green onions
2 cloves garlic
¼ cup olive oil
1 tablespoon fresh lemon juice
1 teaspoon oregano
Salt and pepper to taste

Directions
Place salmon fillets in a glass baking dish side by side, with the skin side down. Pulse herbs, onion, oil, and seasonings in a food processor until well combined. Spread mixture over salmon. Cover and marinate in refrigerator for several hours. Place on preheated grill, skin side down, and cook on high heat for 5–10 minutes until fully cooked.

Yield: Serves 4.

Nutritional information per serving: Calories: 294, Fat: 21g, Carbohydrates: 1g, Fiber: <1g, Protein: 25g.

❖ Asian Grilled Tuna Burgers

Ingredients
16 ounces fresh tuna, ground
1 cup green onions, chopped
½ tablespoon fresh ginger, minced
2 cloves garlic, minced
2 tablespoons soy sauce
½–1 teaspoon crushed red pepper
1 tablespoon fresh lemon juice

Directions
Combine tuna with other ingredients in a large bowl. Mix well and form into patties. Cook on preheated grill on medium-high heat until cooked as desired.

Yield: Serves 4.

Nutritional information per serving: Calories: 167, Fat: 3g, Carbohydrates: 2g, Fiber: <1g, Protein: 30g.

❖ Surprise Pesto Chicken Sandwiches

Ingredients
4 slices focaccia bread
¼ cup pesto sauce
2 tablespoons Jamaican jerk seasoning
1 cup cooked chicken, shredded
½ cup spinach, washed and chopped

Directions
Lightly toast or grill focaccia bread. Spread 1 tablespoon of pesto on each slice of focaccia. Sprinkle with jerk seasoning. Divide chicken into 2 servings and place each serving on 1 slice of focaccia. Top with spinach and the other slice of focaccia.

Yield: Serves 2.

Nutritional information per serving: Calories: 481, Fat: 17g, Carbohydrates: 52g, Fiber: 5g, Protein: 29g.

❖ Mediterranean Chicken with Spinach and Feta

Ingredients
4 cups fresh spinach, chopped
4 chicken breasts, boneless and skinless
1 cup feta cheese, crumbled
1 tablespoon fresh parsley, minced

1 garlic clove, minced
1 tablespoon olive oil
2 tablespoons butter
2 tablespoons all-purpose flour
1 cup chicken stock
½ cup dry white wine
1 teaspoon garlic powder
⅓ cup half-and-half
Salt and pepper to taste

Directions
Place spinach in a saucepan with tight fitted lid. Heat on medium heat until slightly wilted, then drain. Slice the chicken breasts in half almost all the way through to form a pocket. Spread each chicken breast open and cover with waxed paper. Gently hammer each chicken flat with a meat mallet, or use a rolling pin. Remove paper and fill with spinach, feta, parsley, and garlic. Place a toothpick in each breast to seal it. Place olive oil in a large skillet and cook chicken on medium-high heat until cooked through. While chicken is cooking, melt butter on medium heat in a small saucepan. Stir in flour and mix well. Add chicken stock, wine, and garlic powder. Bring to a boil. Pour sauce over chicken and cook for 15–20 minutes as flavors mix. Pour in half-and-half and heat until warmed.

Yield: Serves 4.

Nutritional information per serving: Calories: 500, Fat: 16g, Carbohydrates: 7g, Fiber: 1g, Protein: 44g.

❖ Creamed Chicken Tortilla Bake

Ingredients
6 6-inch flour tortillas
1 tablespoon olive oil
½ cup onion, diced
1 red pepper, diced
2 cloves garlic, minced
½ teaspoon crushed red pepper
1 10-ounce can low-fat cream of mushroom soup

1 15-ounce can pinto beans, drained and rinsed
2 tablespoons fresh cilantro, chopped
6 ounces sour cream
1 teaspoon garlic powder
2 cups boneless chicken, cooked, chopped
1 tomato, deseeded, diced
8 ounces Monterey Jack cheese and/or cheddar cheese, shredded
Salt and pepper to taste

Directions
Cut tortillas into 2-inch-wide strips and set aside. Heat olive oil in a large pan and cook onion and red pepper for 5–6 minutes until vegetables begin to soften. Stir in garlic and crushed red pepper. Turn off heat. Combine soup, beans, cilantro, sour cream, and garlic powder in a large mixing bowl. Fold in chicken, tomato, and vegetables. Add salt and pepper to taste. Stir to combine. Pour half of chicken mixture into a large glass pan. Layer half of tortilla strips over mixture. Pour the rest of the chicken mixture into the pan. Top with remaining tortilla strips. Cover dish with tomatoes and shredded cheese. Cover with foil and bake at 375 degrees for 30 minutes. Remove foil and bake an additional 15 minutes or until moisture is absorbed.

Yield: Serves 8.

Nutritional information per serving: Calories: 359, Fat: 17g,
    Carbohydrates: 28g, Fiber: 5g, Protein: 24g.

❖ Zesty Quesadillas

Ingredients
1 tablespoon olive oil
1 small yellow onion, diced
2 garlic cloves, minced
2 cups fresh spinach, chopped
½ cup feta cheese
4 ounces Neufchatel cheese
1 tablespoon fresh lemon juice
¼ teaspoon ground cumin

2 tablespoons fresh cilantro
½ teaspoon ground nutmeg
¼ teaspoon ground cinnamon
4 6-inch wheat tortillas
Salt and pepper to taste

Directions
Heat olive oil in a medium skillet. Cook onion until translucent. Stir in garlic and spinach and cook 2–3 minutes. Drain on paper towels and set aside. Combine feta cheese, Neufchatel cheese, lemon juice, cumin, cilantro, nutmeg, and cinnamon in a large bowl. Add salt and pepper. Stir well. Fold spinach and onions into mixture. Quarter mixture and spoon onto one side of each tortilla. Fold tortilla in half to form quesadilla. Spread on a pan and bake at 350 degrees for 15 minutes or until toasted, flipping halfway through.

Yield: Serves 4.

Nutritional information per serving: Calories: 266, Fat: 13g, Carbohydrates: 19g, Fiber: 3g, Protein: 6g.

❖ Pastitsio

Ingredients
16 ounces penne pasta
2 tablespoons olive oil
1 pound lean ground beef or soy beef substitute
1 large onion, diced
2 tablespoons tomato paste
1 28-ounce can tomato sauce
2 tablespoons water
⅓ cup ricotta cheese
⅓ cup low-fat sour cream
¼ cup freshly grated Parmesan
¼ teaspoon ground cinnamon
½ teaspoon fresh ground nutmeg
2 tablespoons butter
⅔ cup half-and-half
Salt and pepper to taste

Directions
Boil water in a large saucepan and cook penne pasta until al dente. Drain and set aside. While pasta is cooking, add olive oil to a large sauté pan. Cook beef and onion in oil on medium-high heat until golden brown. Add tomato paste, tomato sauce, and water to beef and stir well to combine. Add salt and pepper to taste. Spread beef and tomato mixture in a large glass baking dish. In a large bowl, combine penne pasta with ricotta, sour cream, Parmesan, cinnamon, and nutmeg. Mix well and spread over the meat mixture. In a small saucepan, heat butter and half-and-half on medium heat and cook just to a boil. Pour half-and-half and butter over the pasta in the dish. Cover with foil and bake at 350 degrees for 30 minutes. Remove foil and bake 10 minutes more, until moisture is mostly absorbed.

Yield: Serves 8.

Nutritional information per serving: Calories: 426, Fat: 14g,
    Carbohydrates: 56g, Fiber: 7g, Protein: 22g.

❖ Beef Stroganoff

Ingredients
2 tablespoons olive oil
1 pound ground beef or soy beef substitute
1 large onion, diced
8 ounces sliced mushrooms
2 cloves garlic, minced
2 tablespoons flour
1 teaspoon garlic powder
1 teaspoon onion powder
Dash of nutmeg
1 cup vegetable broth
1 tablespoon Worcestershire sauce
12 ounces light sour cream
16 ounces egg noodles, cooked according to package directions
Salt and pepper to taste

Directions
Heat 1 tablespoon olive oil in a large sauté pan and add beef. Cook on medium high heat until cooked through. Set aside. In a large saucepan

heat 1 tablespoon olive oil and add onions, mushrooms, and garlic. Cook on medium heat for several minutes. Stir in beef. Cook 5 minutes. Add flour, garlic powder, onion powder, and nutmeg. Cook another 5 minutes. Stir in vegetable broth and Worcestershire sauce. Cook 10 minutes. Add sour cream, then salt and pepper. Stir to combine. Serve over egg noodles.

Yield: Serves 8.

Nutritional information per serving: Calories: 386, Fat: 12g,
    Carbohydrates: 46g, Fiber: 2g, Protein: 25g.

❖ Baked Spaghetti

Ingredients
8 ounces spaghetti
2 tablespoons olive oil
1 pound lean ground beef or soy beef substitute
1 medium onion, chopped
2 cloves garlic, minced
1 28-ounce can tomato sauce
2 tablespoons tomato paste
1 tablespoon sugar
1 tablespoon onion powder
1 tablespoon garlic powder
1 teaspoon dried rosemary, crushed
1 teaspoon dried oregano
1 egg
1 tablespoon olive oil
¾ cup ricotta cheese
½ cup Parmesan cheese, grated
¾ cup mozzarella cheese, grated
Salt and pepper to taste

Directions
Prepare spaghetti according to package directions. Drain and set aside. Heat 2 tablespoons olive oil in a large skillet and cook beef for several minutes. Add onion and garlic and stir, cooking until beef is cooked

through. Pour tomato sauce and tomato paste into the skillet and stir well. Add sugar, herbs, and salt and pepper. Cook for 10 minutes and set aside. Beat egg with a fork. Stir egg and 1 tablespoon olive oil into spaghetti noodles and spread noodles over the bottom of a large baking dish. Spread ricotta cheese on top. Pour sauce over the ricotta cheese and top with grated mozzarella. Cover with foil and cook at 350 degrees for 25 minutes until moisture is absorbed. Remove foil and cook an additional 10 minutes until cheese is golden brown.

Yield: Serves 6.

Nutritional information per serving: Calories: 515, Fat: 21g, Carbohydrates: 45g, Fiber: 6g, Protein: 34g.

❖ Sweet and Sour Meatballs

Ingredients
1 teaspoon canola oil
1 small green pepper, finely diced
1 clove garlic, minced
1 15-ounce can diced pineapple in fruit juice
¼ cup light corn syrup
1 tablespoon white vinegar
1 tablespoon ketchup
1 tablespoon soy sauce
1 tablespoon cornstarch
1 tablespoon water
1 pound meatballs (or soy meatball substitute), cooked

Directions
Heat oil in a small saucepan and add green pepper and garlic. Cook on medium heat for several minutes until vegetables begin to soften. Pour in the rest of the ingredients, except for the meatballs. Stir well to combine. Bring to a boil, then turn down heat and simmer for 3–4 minutes, stirring well. Add cooked meatballs to pot and simmer on low heat for 10 minutes until flavors are absorbed. Serve over rice or egg noodles.

Yield: Serves 4.

Nutritional information per serving: Calories: 274, Fat: 7g,
    Carbohydrates: 30g, Fiber: 2g, Protein: 24g.

✤ Eggs Benedict

Ingredients
4 eggs
1 teaspoon distilled white vinegar
4 slices cooked ham
2 English muffins, halved
1 package Hollandaise sauce
1 tablespoon fresh tarragon, chopped
Salt and pepper to taste

Directions
Fill a large saucepot with 2 inches of water and bring to a boil. Pour in
vinegar and turn down heat to a low simmer. Crack eggs into a small glass.
With a quick turn of the hand, pour an egg into the water. Continue with
each egg and cook eggs for 3–5 minutes. Carefully remove each egg with a
slotted spoon and drain on paper towels. (Eggs should be firm but runny
in the middle.) Heat ham and toast English muffins. Prepare Hollandaise
sauce according to package directions. Place ham and egg over each
muffin and spoon Hollandaise sauce on top. Sprinkle with fresh tarragon
and salt and pepper.

Yield: Serves 4.

Nutritional information per serving: Calories: 226, Fat: 11g,
    Carbohydrates: 17g, Fiber: 1g, Protein: 15g.

✤ Vegetarian Sausage and Pepperoni Pizza

Ingredients
2 tablespoons olive oil
6 ounces soy sausage substitute
4 ounces soy pepperoni substitute
2 cloves garlic, minced

⅓ cup yellow onion, diced
1 teaspoon oregano
½ teaspoon salt
½ teaspoon pepper
12 ounces mozzarella (or soy mozzarella) cheese, shredded
1 large prepared pizza crust, room temperature
8-ounce can tomato sauce

Directions
Heat olive oil in a small sauté pan, add soy sausage and pepperoni and cook on medium-high heat for several minutes, stirring occasionally. Add garlic, onion, oregano, and salt and pepper, and stir again, heating until sausage and pepperoni are browned. Spread tomato sauce over pizza crust. Layer meat and onion mixture on top. Sprinkle with mozzarella cheese. Bake at 450 degrees for 10–15 minutes until cheese is browned and crust is cooked through.

Yield: Serves 4.

Nutritional information per serving: Calories: 610, Fat: 24g,
    Carbohydrates: 48g, Fiber: 6g, Protein: 45g.

VEGETABLES

✤ Asparagus with Lemon and Parmesan

Ingredients
20 large stalks of asparagus
2 tablespoons fresh lemon juice
¼ cup vegetable broth
1 tablespoon fresh tarragon, chopped
1 clove garlic, minced
4 tablespoons freshly grated Parmesan cheese

Directions
Cut off the tough parts of the asparagus and discard. Pour lemon juice, broth, tarragon, and garlic in a large saucepan. Stir and bring to a boil, cooking 2 minutes as flavors mingle. Arrange asparagus tips in a single

layer in the pot and cover, cooking just until tender. Drain. Sprinkle with Parmesan cheese just before serving.

Yield: Serves 3.

Nutritional information per serving: Calories: 62, Fat: <1g, Carbohydrates: 7g, Fiber: 3g, Protein: 4g.

❖ Rice and Peas

Ingredients
8 ounces canned pigeon peas
½ cup coconut milk
1 tablespoon fresh thyme
1 cup brown rice, cooked
Hot sauce, optional

Directions
Place pigeon peas in a small saucepan on medium heat. Stir in coconut milk and thyme. Cook for 10–15 minutes as flavors blend. Serve over rice and season with hot sauce.

Yield: Serves 3.

Nutritional information per serving: Calories: 214, Fat: 9g, Carbohydrates: 29g, Fiber: 5g, Protein: 6g.

❖ Mother Mac's Elegant Carrots

Ingredients
1 tablespoon canola oil
1 medium onion, chopped fine
4 cups carrots, julienned
¼ cup orange juice
1 tablespoon brown sugar
16 ounces light sour cream
1 tablespoon sugar
1 cup sharp cheddar cheese, shredded

Directions
Heat canola oil in a large saucepan and add onion and carrots. Cook for 5 minutes until vegetables begin to soften. Pour orange juice and brown sugar over vegetables. Cover and cook on medium-low heat for 15 minutes as carrots continue to soften. Pour carrots into a large glass baking dish. Combine sour cream and sugar in a small bowl. Pour over carrots and top with shredded cheese. Cover and bake at 350 degrees for 20 minutes.

Yield: Serves 10.

Nutritional information per serving: Calories: 205, Fat: 11g,
    Carbohydrates: 11g, Fiber: 1g, Protein: 12g.

✤ Broccoli Quiche

Ingredients
⅔ cup broccoli florets, chopped
6 ounces cheddar cheese, shredded
1 prepared piecrust
4 eggs, beaten with fork
1 cup half-and-half
¼ cup onions, diced
½ teaspoon dried basil
½ teaspoon dried oregano
2 tomatoes, deseeded and thinly sliced
Salt and pepper to taste

Directions
Layer broccoli and cheese in the piecrust. Beat eggs with fork and stir in half-and-half, onions, and herbs. Pour over broccoli and cheese. Bake at 350 degrees for 45 minutes. Lay tomatoes on top of the quiche and broil for 2–3 minutes until browned.

Yield: Serves 8.

Nutritional information per serving: Calories: 251, Fat: 18g,
    Carbohydrates: 12g, Fiber: 1g, Protein: 11g.

❖ Colorful Roasted Peppers

Ingredients
2 tablespoons olive oil
2 large red peppers, deseeded, cut in half
1 small yellow squash, diced
1 small zucchini squash, diced
½ cup red onion, diced
½ cup portabella mushrooms, sliced
2 cloves garlic, minced
6 ounces Monterey Jack with pepper cheese, shredded
2 tablespoons Jamaican jerk marinade or jerk seasoning
½ teaspoon salt

Directions
Grease inside and outside of red peppers with 1 tablespoon olive oil. Place red peppers side by side in a small pan. Roast at 450 degrees for 3–4 minutes until red peppers begin to soften and blacken. Set aside. In a small saucepan, combine 1 tablespoon olive oil with vegetables and salt and cook on medium heat for 5 minutes until vegetables are crisp-tender. Turn off heat. Divide cheese into four parts. Spoon jerk marinade and 1 tablespoon of cheese into the bottom of each pepper. Divide vegetables and spoon into peppers. Top with the remaining cheese. Cover pan with foil and bake peppers at 400 degrees for 10 minutes. Remove foil and bake an additional 5 minutes or until cheese is melted and lightly browned.

Yield: Serves 4.

Nutritional information per serving: Calories: 277, Fat: 20g,
    Carbohydrates: 13g, Fiber: 4g, Protein: 13g.

❖ Summer Squash Gratin

Ingredients
2 tablespoons butter
2 large yellow squash, cut in half-circles
2 large zucchini squash, cut into half-circles

1 small yellow onion, diced
4 garlic cloves, minced
1½ cups bread crumbs
1 egg
½ cup half-and-half
1 cup cheddar cheese, grated
1 teaspoon dried oregano
½ teaspoon crushed dried thyme
Salt and pepper to taste

Directions
Place 2 tablespoons butter in a large sauté pan with the squash, onion, and garlic. Cook for several minutes until vegetables are tender. Set aside. In a large bowl, combine ½ cup bread crumbs, egg, half-and-half, and ½ cup of cheddar cheese. Fold in vegetables and stir gently. Add salt and pepper to taste. Turn mixture into a glass baking dish. Top with remaining bread crumbs and cheddar cheese and cover with foil. Bake at 375 degrees for 30 minutes. Remove foil and bake for 10 minutes until casserole is set.

Yield: Serves 8.

Nutritional information per serving: Calories: 227, Fat: 15g,
    Carbohydrates: 14g, Fiber: 3g, Protein: 11g.

❖ Creamy Artichoke Dip

Ingredients
2 tablespoons canola oil
1 large bunch green onions, sliced
6 cloves garlic, minced
2 cups fresh spinach, chopped
10 ounces artichoke hearts, jarred or frozen (if frozen, thaw before preparing), chopped
8 ounces Neufchatel cream cheese, cut into small cubes
16 ounces low-fat sour cream
8 ounces sharp cheddar cheese
1 large round loaf of bread

Directions

Sauté green onions and garlic in the canola oil. Cook on medium-high heat until softened. Stir in spinach and cover, steaming for several minutes until spinach is wilted. Drain liquid from spinach mixture. Combine vegetables with all other ingredients. Mix well. Cut a large hole in the top of the loaf of bread. Scoop out the inside of the bread loaf, leaving the round crust intact. Pour into bread loaf and wrap in aluminum foil. Bake at 400 degrees for 2 hours until cheese mixture is hot and creamy. Serve with crackers, toasted baguette, or raw vegetables.

Yield: Serves 12.

Nutritional information per serving: Calories: 200, Fat: 15g,
    Carbohydrates: 7g, Fiber: 1g, Protein: 11g.

❖ Hearty Vegetable Spread

Ingredients
1 tablespoon olive oil
1 cup yellow onion
3 cloves garlic, minced
1 cup broccoli
1 large zucchini
½ cup mushrooms
⅔ cup artichoke hearts
6 ounces cream cheese, softened
8 ounces sour cream
⅔ cup chopped walnuts
1 cup bread crumbs
Salt and pepper to taste

Directions

Chop all vegetables into very small uniform pieces. Pour olive oil in a large sauté pan and add onions. Cook at medium-high heat for several minutes until onions are golden. Turn heat down to medium and add garlic, broccoli, zucchini, mushrooms, and artichokes. Cook for several minutes until vegetables are crisp-tender. Set aside to cool. In a mixing bowl, combine cream cheese, sour cream, and bread crumbs. Stir well.

Stir in walnuts and gently fold in vegetables. Pour into a greased glass baking dish and cover with foil. Bake at 350 degrees for 45 minutes. Remove foil and cook for several minutes more until creamy. Serve warm with crackers or toasted bread.

Yield: Serves 12.

Nutritional information per serving: Calories: 166, Fat: 12g, Carbohydrates: 9g, Fiber: 2g, Protein: 7g.

❖ Spinach and Corn Pastry

Ingredients
1 tablespoon olive oil
¼ cup yellow onion
2 cloves garlic, minced
3 cups fresh spinach, washed and chopped
9 frozen puff pastry sheets, thawed
½ cup mozzarella cheese, grated
¼ cup freshly grated Parmesan
½ cup canned or fresh yellow corn
1 egg white, beaten
Salt and pepper to taste

Directions
Heat olive oil, onion, and garlic in a medium saucepan on medium heat. Cook for several minutes until onion is translucent. Stir in spinach and cover, cooking for 2–3 minutes until spinach is wilted. Drain any liquid out and set aside. In a mixing bowl, combine corn with cheeses and fold in spinach mixture. Lay out pastry sheets on top of each other and brush top sheet with egg white. Spread cheese and vegetable mixture evenly over pastry. Carefully roll pastry into a log. Cut into 12 slices and place together on a large baking sheet. Cook at 400 degrees for 15 minutes until golden.

Yield: Serves 6.

Nutritional information per serving: Calories: 208, Fat: 7g, Carbohydrates: 25g, Fiber: 2g, Protein: 11g.

❖ Roasted Parsnips

Ingredients
2 16-ounce packages of parsnips, diced into 1-inch cubes
1 red onion, sliced
1–2 tablespoons fresh rosemary, chopped
1 tablespoon Worcestershire sauce
¼ cup balsamic vinegar
1 tablespoon brown sugar
2 tablespoons olive oil
Salt and pepper to taste

Directions
Combine parsnips and onion with rosemary, Worcestershire sauce, vinegar, and brown sugar. Mix well, cover, and refrigerate for 4 hours or overnight, mixing occasionally. Preheat oven to 450 degrees. Coat a roasting pan with olive oil. Remove parsnips from marinade and spread in roasting pan. Add salt and pepper to taste. Cook for 30 minutes or until parsnips are softened and cooked through.

Yield: Serves 6.

Nutritional information per serving: Calories: 89, Fat: 5g, Carbohydrates: 12g, Fiber: 2g, Protein: 1g.

❖ Indian Curried Sweet Potato

Ingredients
2 tablespoons canola oil
1 cup sweet potato, diced
1 small yellow onion, diced
2 cloves garlic, minced
8 ounces light coconut milk
¼ teaspoon ground cumin
½ teaspoon ground coriander
1 teaspoon chili powder
1 cup cooked rice

Directions
Heat oil in a saucepan. Heat sweet potato on medium heat, stirring occasionally. Cover and steam for 5–10 minutes until sweet potato softens. (Add 1 tablespoon of water at a time if sweet potatoes start to brown too quickly.) Add onions and garlic and cook on medium heat for several minutes until onions are translucent. Add coconut milk and spices. Let simmer on medium-low heat for 5–10 minutes as flavors combine. Serve over cooked rice.

Yield: Serves 4.

Nutritional information per serving: Calories: 270, Fat: 19g, Carbohydrates: 24g, Fiber: 2g, Protein: 3g.

❖ Mom's Baked Beans

Ingredients
1 28-ounce can vegetarian baked beans
8 ounces frozen lima beans
1 15-ounce can kidney beans
1 white onion, diced
½ cup diced green pepper
2 tablespoons vinegar
2 tablespoons brown sugar
¼ cup spicy brown mustard
¼ cup ketchup

Directions
Combine all ingredients in a large glass pan. Bake at 350 degrees for 45 minutes or until bubbly.

Yield: Serves 10.

Nutritional information per serving: Calories: 184, Fat: 1g, Carbohydrates: 37g, Fiber: 9g, Protein: 9g.

DESERTS

✤ Fried Bananas

Ingredients
3 large ripe bananas
¼ cup coconut milk
2 tablespoons canola oil
Honey, powdered sugar (optional)

Directions
Place oil in a small sauté pan on medium heat. Peel bananas and slice four times diagonally, creating thick slices. Dip bananas in the coconut milk and place in oil, frying for several minutes until golden brown. Do not overcook. Drizzle with honey and sprinkle with powdered sugar if desired.

Yield: Serves 3.

Nutritional information per serving: Calories: 222, Fat: 14g, Carbohydrates: 28g, Fiber: 1g, Protein: 1g.

✤ Sweet Strawberry Pie

Ingredients
1 graham cracker piecrust
1 2.5-ounce package sugar-free strawberry gelatin
2 cups thinly sliced strawberries
8 ounces Neufchatel cheese, softened
½ cup powdered sugar
Whipped cream (optional)

Directions
Prepare gelatin according to package directions. Refrigerate gelatin for 1 hour until it starts to thicken. Pour strawberries into gelatin and stir. Pour gelatin mixture into the graham cracker crust. Refrigerate until pie is firm. Combine Neufchatel cheese and powdered sugar in a mixing bowl. Beat well for several minutes. Spread cream cheese mixture over pie and refrigerate again for several hours. Top with whipped cream before serving, if desired.

Yield: Serves 8.

Nutritional information per serving: Calories: 260, Fat: 14g,
    Carbohydrates: 31g, Fiber: 1g, Protein: 4g.

❖ Peanut Butter Cookies

Ingredients
1½ cups unbleached flour
½ teaspoon baking soda
½ teaspoon salt
½ cup brown sugar
½ cup white sugar
¾ cup peanut butter
½ cup butter, softened
1 teaspoon vanilla extract

Directions
Grease several cookie sheets. Sift flour, baking soda, and salt into a small
bowl. In a large mixing bowl, cream sugars, peanut butter, and butter. Stir
in the dry ingredients in small batches. Stir in vanilla. Scoop up 1
tablespoon of the dough at a time, forming a ball and then flattening it
slightly onto the greased pan. Bake at 350 degrees for 12–15 minutes
until cookies are done. Allow to cool before serving.

Yield: 20 cookies.

Nutritional information per serving: Calories: 162, Fat: 9g, Carbohydrates:
    20g, Fiber: 1g, Protein: 5g.

❖ Fruit and Nut Cake

Ingredients
3 cups white flour
2 teaspoons baking soda
½ teaspoon salt
3 eggs

2 cups white sugar
1¼ cups canola oil
1½ teaspoons vanilla
1 teaspoon ground cinnamon
1 cup crushed pineapple, drained
¾ cup pecans, chopped finely
¼ cup walnuts, chopped finely
2 large bananas, finely chopped (use bananas that are just ripe)

LEMON FROSTING:
Ingredients
16 ounces low-fat cream cheese, softened
½ cup butter, softened
4 cups powdered sugar
2 teaspoons vanilla
Juice from 1 lemon

Directions
Grease and flour three 9-inch round pans. Sift flour, baking soda, and salt together in a small bowl. Whisk eggs together in a small bowl. In a large mixing bowl, combine sugar, oil, vanilla, and cinnamon. Mix well, then add eggs, pineapple, and nuts. Mix again and fold in bananas. Pour batter into pans and bake at 350 degrees for 25–30 minutes or until done. Test with toothpick. Allow cakes to cool. While cakes are baking, mix frosting ingredients until creamy and smooth. After cakes are cool, frost them with the icing. Stack one on top of the other and smooth icing over edges.

Yield: Serves 20.

Nutritional information per serving: Calories: 523, Fat: 28g, Carbohydrates: 64g, Fiber: 1g, Protein: 5g.

CHAPTER 8

Bone-Building Exercises

Use the following stretches, range-of-motion, and isometric or strength-ening exercises to supplement your Bone-Building Workout (Step 2).

Stretching Exercises

Stretch throughout the day to keep muscles limber and flexible. Stretch-ing helps to ease stiffness and allows you to be more active. Being flexible helps to prevent falls, a major cause of hip fracture.

Chest and Mid-Back
Place a broom handle or a long pole behind your back and across your shoulders with your hands supporting the long handle or pole at each end. Then slowly rotate your torso to the left; repeat this movement in the opposite direction. (Figure 8.1)

Shoulders
Hold a broom handle or long pole with both hands over your head and slowly stretch from side to side like a pendulum several times. Then place the handle or pole at shoulder level in front of you and gently turn to the right as far as is comfortable, then to the left. Repeat several times. (Fig-ure 8.2)

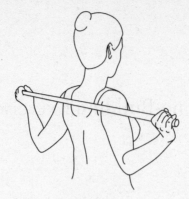

Figure 8.1

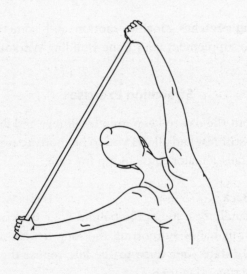

Figure 8.2

Neck

Place one hand on the side of your head just above the ear and gently push as if you are trying to place your ear on your shoulder. Gradually build pressure while allowing no movement to occur. Hold and then relax. (Figure 8.3)

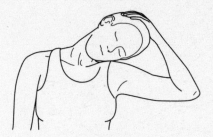

Figure 8.3

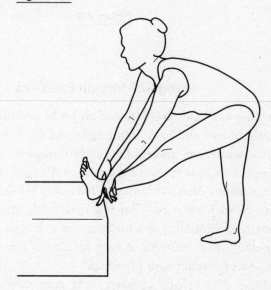

Figure 8.4

Legs and Hamstrings
Stand upright and put foot on bench (or step). Slowly bend forward at the hip while keeping your back straight. Alternate to the other leg and repeat exercise. You should feel the stretch behind your thigh. (Figure 8.4)

Back
This exercise will help keep your posture straight and alleviate stress on the back and hips. Lie on your back with your knees bent and feet flat on the floor and hip-width apart. While contracting your abdominal muscles, press your lower back against the floor. You will feel your pelvis rock (tilt) toward your shoulders. The bottom of your buttocks and your pelvis will come slightly off the floor during the action. (Figure 8.5)

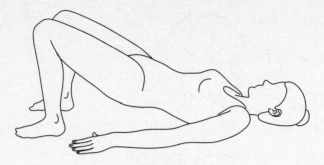

Figure 8.5

Range-of-Motion Exercises

The following exercises are designed to build flexibility and strength in the neck, shoulders, and back. Being agile and flexible helps you to maintain balance, which can prevent falls and subsequent fractures.

It is important to work toward a goal of doing these exercises twice a day, 20 repetitions each. At first, you may only be able to do one to two repetitions of each exercise. That is a reasonable start. However, as you gain strength and mobility, gradually increase as you can and move into the twice-daily, 20 repetitions of each routine. If you have any pain, stop the exercise and contact your physician.

Sometimes it is helpful to have some gentle assistance from a family member or friend. Your physician or physical therapist can show you how.

A word of caution: Do not hold your breath while performing any exercise. If you feel pain with any of the suggested exercises, stop the exercise and discuss this with your physician.

Neck Range-of-Motion Exercises

It is important to build strength in the neck as well as improve mobility and flexibility. These range-of-motion exercises will enable your body to perform more effectively. While flexion should be done standing, the rest of the neck exercises can be performed sitting or standing, whichever is more comfortable for you.

Flexion

While standing, look down and bend your chin forward to the chest. If you feel stiffness or pain, do not force the movement. Go as far as you can without straining yourself. If you have pain with this or any exercise, stop until you have talked to your physician or physical therapist.

Extension

Look up and bend your head back as far as possible without forcing any movement.

Lateral Flexion

Tilt your left ear to your left shoulder (but do not raise the shoulder). If you feel pain or resistance, do not force the motion.

Now tilt the ear to the right shoulder just as you did for the left ear. (Figure 8.6).

Rotation

Turn to look over your left shoulder. Try to make your chin even with your shoulder. Go as far as is comfortable, but do not force the movement.

Now turn and look over your right shoulder, as you did with the left.

Neck Isometric Exercises

Neck isometric exercises are more advanced exercises to help strengthen the muscles of the neck. Try these gently and gradually after range-of-motion of your neck is improved as much as possible. Again, do not hold your breath.

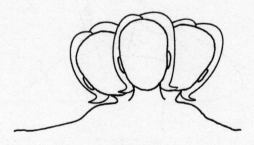

Figure 8.6

Lateral flexion

Isometric Flexion

Place hand on your forehead. Try to look down while resisting the motion with your hand. Hold for 6 seconds. Count out loud.

Isometric Extension

Place your hands on the back of your head. Try to look up and back while resisting the motion with your hands. Hold for 6 seconds. Count out loud.

Isometric Lateral Flexion

Start with your head straight. Place your left hand just above your left ear. Try to tilt your head to the left but resist the motion with your left hand. Hold for 6 seconds. Count out loud.

Now place your right hand just above your right ear. Try to tilt your head to the right but resist the movement with your right hand. Hold for 6 seconds. Count out loud. (Figure 8.7.)

Isometric Rotation

Place your left hand above your ear and near your left forehead. Now try to look over your left shoulder, but resist the motion with your left hand. The hand should not be placed on the jaw. Hold for 6 seconds. Count out loud.

Place your right hand above your ear and near your right forehead. Now try to look over your right shoulder but resist the motion with your right hand. Hold for 6 seconds. Count out loud.

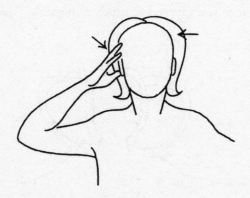

Figure 8.7

Isometric lateral flexion

Shoulder Range-of-Motion Exercises

The following five range-of-motion exercises will increase the flexibility of the shoulders and arms. Increasing the number of exercises can increase the strength of the arms.

Shoulder External Rotation

This exercise increases the motion you use to comb your hair. You may sit, stand, or lie down to do these exercises.

Clasp your hands behind your head. Pull your elbows together until they are as close as possible in front of your chin. Separate the elbows to the side as much as possible.

Repeat this, gradually increasing to 5, then 10, then up to 20 repetitions. You may repeat these 2 or 3 times daily.

Shoulder Internal Rotation

Shoulder internal rotation increases the flexibility of the shoulders. Using the same motions women use to fasten a bra in the back or men use to put a wallet in a back pocket, move your arms in the position as shown in Figure 8.8. This exercise is best done standing and is often done in the shower using a washcloth to wash your upper back or a towel to dry it.

Put your hand behind your back. Then put the other hand behind your back and cross the wrist as shown in the picture. Return the hands to rest at your side.

Repeat this, gradually increasing to 5, then 10, then up to 20 repetitions. Repeat twice daily.

Shoulder Flexion

Shoulder flexion holds both arms down at your sides. Raise the left arm straight up and reach overhead toward the ceiling. Now do the same with the right arm. Continue this motion as you alternate left-right-left-right. Repeat this, gradually increasing to 5, then 10, then up to 20 repetitions, and repeat the exercise twice daily.

Shoulder Adduction

Raise both arms straight out away from your sides, and then raise each arm overhead toward the ceiling and up above your head. Do this with your palm up or palm down.

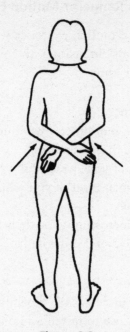

Figure 8.8

Shoulder internal rotation

If this exercise is painful while sitting or standing, you can also do it while lying on your bed. Use a stick (a broom handle will do) as you raise your arms, hold the stick with both hands and keep the arms straight, up over your head as far as possible. If you have pain, the strength of the less painful arm will help the painful arm move more easily.

Repeat this exercise, gradually increasing to 5, then 10, then 20 repetitions 2 or 3 times a day.

Once you have mastered the exercise, go to the second part. This involves raising your arms out to the side, one a time, then slowly making big circles.

Repeat this exercise, gradually increasing to 5, then 10, then 20 repetitions 2 or 3 times a day.

Shoulder Girdle Rotation

This exercise can be done in a sitting or standing position and is fun to do during the day to relieve neck and shoulder tension and maintain shoulder girdle flexibility.

Roll shoulders in a forward circle; raise shoulders toward the ears in a shrugging motion. Roll shoulders back and chest out as in a military stance. Lower the shoulders and bring the shoulders forward. Think of it as a simple shoulder roll in a circle. Now reverse the process, rolling your shoulder girdle in a backward circle.

Repeat this exercise, gradually increasing to 5, then 10, then 20 repetitions 2 or 3 times a day if possible.

Back Exercises

Back exercises help to strengthen the muscles supporting the spine, which is an important part of your osteopenia prevention program.

As you do the following strengthening exercises, it is very important that you breathe properly while holding the position. Counting to 6 aloud will enable you to do this easily. If you experience shortness of breath, stop and talk to your doctor or physical therapist.

Cheek to Cheek

This is a convenient exercise because you can do it anywhere, anytime, and practically in any position. It strengthens the muscles of the buttocks that help support the back and the legs. When sitting, you will actually rise up out of the chair because of the contraction of the muscle groups in the buttocks.

Press your buttocks together and hold for a 6-second count. Relax and repeat. Gradually increase to 5, then 10, then 20 repetitions. Repeat 2 times daily.

Do this exercise frequently during the day.

Pelvic Tilt

This is one of the best exercises you can do to strengthen your abdominal muscles, which in turn help support your back. Strong backs help you to have good posture. This exercise will also help tone your stomach muscles. Do this exercise lying on your back in bed or on the floor, whichever is more comfortable.

Relax and raise your arms above your head. Keep your knees bent. Now comes the tricky part! Tighten the muscles of your lower abdomen and your buttocks at the same time to flatten your back against the floor or bed. Hold the flat-back position for a 6-second count. Now relax and repeat.

Repeat this exercise 2 or 3 times to start and work gradually to 5, then 10, then 20 repetitions.

If you have trouble, contact your physical therapist or physician and have them demonstrate the exercise. This may be particularly necessary if you want to do this exercise standing up or sitting in a chair.

Bridging

This exercise strengthens the muscles in the back. Lie on your back on the floor or in bed and bend (flex) your hips and knees. Now lift your hips and buttocks off the bed or floor 4 to 6 inches, forcing the small of the back out flat; and tighten the buttock and hip muscles to maintain this position. Hold this position for a count of 6 seconds. Now, relax and lower your hips and buttocks to the floor or bed.

Repeat this exercise, gradually increasing up to 5, then 10, then 20 repetitions as tolerated. Repeat this twice daily if possible. (Figure 8.9)

Partial Sit-Up

This is one of the more vigorous exercises. Its purpose is to build abdominal strength to give the back greater support.

To do this exercise lie on your bed or on the floor, whichever is more comfortable.

Lie on your back with your knees bent. Raise your head and shoulder blades off the floor or bed. Hold that position for a 6-second count. Slowly return to the beginning position of lying on your back. Repeat.

Start this exercise slowly with 1 or 2 repetitions until your body adjusts. Gradually increase to 5, then 10 repetitions. (Figure 8.10)

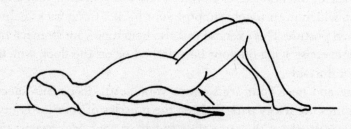

Figure 8.9

A bridging exercise

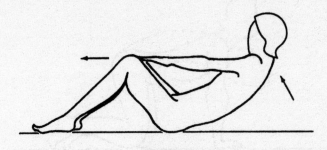

Figure 8.10

A partial sit-up exercise

Back Extension

For this exercise to strengthen the back muscles, lie on your bed or on the floor in a prone (stomach down) position. A pillow may be used under the stomach to help make this position more comfortable.

Raise your head, arms, and legs off the floor. Do not bend your knees. This must be done with your body straight in extension. Hold for 6 seconds while you count out loud. Relax and repeat.

Gradually increase to 5, then 10 repetitions. If you experience discomfort, check with your physician or physical therapist before you continue.

Cat Camel

Do not do this exercise for strengthening the back muscles if you have very painful knees, ankles, or hands since it places pressure on these areas.

The position for this exercise is a crawling position. Hands must be directly under your shoulders. Take a deep breath and arch your back as a frightened cat does, lowering your head. Hold that position while you count 6 seconds out loud. Now exhale and drop the arched back slowly, raising your head.

Start this exercise slowly with 1 or 2 repetitions. Increase to 5 and then 10 repetitions if possible. (Figure 8.11)

Wall Push

This exercise is good for the back because it encourages the body extension positions.

Stand spread eagle with your back against a solid wall. Now arch your back inward slowly.

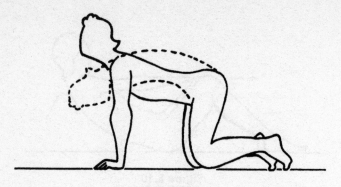

Figure 8.11

Cat camel exercise

Gradually increase repetitions from 1 to 5 or more. This exercise is fun because you can do it any time you feel you need a good body stretch. Repeat twice daily.

Back Flexibility
Lie on your back on the floor with knees bent and feet flat on the floor. Raise hands toward the ceiling. Now move arms and turn the head to the right, while the knees move to the left. Reverse the above, then repeat. Gradually increase to 5 and then 10 repetitions daily.

Bicycling
Lying on your back, move your feet and legs in the air as if you were riding a bicycle. Count to 6, and relax. Repeat, and then gradually increase to 5 and then 10 repetitions once or twice daily if tolerated.

Hip Exercises

These exercises are actually good not only for the hips but for the back and the knees. You can do these exercises on the floor or in bed, but don't do them if you have had a hip or knee total joint replacement.

Flexion
Bend the left knee to the chest, and then bend the right knee to the chest. If needed, you can help by using your hands to help bend the knee.

Repeat, alternating left and right knees. Try to increase to 5, then 10, then up to 20 repetitions, twice daily.

Pull both knees to the chest at the same time. Hold this position for 6 seconds and then slowly rock from side to side while holding the knees. Gently let your legs down. Repeat, gradually increasing to 5, then 10, then 20 repetitions, twice daily. (Figure 8.12)

Adduction

This can be done lying on the floor or in bed. While lying on your back (with knee straight or slightly bent), slide the left leg out to the side then return to the starting position. Now do the same movement with the right leg. Gradually increase to 5, then 10, then 20 repetitions for each leg, twice daily.

Extension

This can be done lying on your stomach on the floor or in bed. Keep the knee straight and lift your left thigh straight up off the floor about 8 inches. Hold this position while you count to 6. Repeat with the right leg, then alternate legs and gradually increase to 5, then 10, then 20 repetitions, twice daily. If there is severe pain, stop until you talk to your doctor. (Figure 8.13)

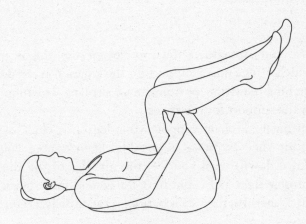

Figure 8.12

Hip flexion

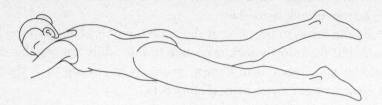

Figure 8.13

Hip extension

Rotation

Lie on your back on the floor or in bed. With your knees straight, turn your knees in and touch your toes together. Now turn the knees out. Repeat this, gradually increasing to 5, then 10, then 20 repetitions, twice daily.

Knee and Leg Exercises

The following knee and leg exercises will help you to support your skeleton and avoid falls. Be sure to do these exercises regularly as part of your plan to prevent fractures.

Extension

This exercise can strengthen the muscles of the thighs (quadriceps muscles), which offer a major support for the knees. You can do this while reading, watching television, or riding in an airplane. The more you do it, the stronger the support for the knees.

While sitting in a chair, support your leg on a chair or table and straighten your knee as much as possible. Then tighten your kneecap (push the knee down) until you feel the muscles of the thigh tighten. Keep that muscle tight and count to 6. Relax, and then repeat, gradually increasing to 5, then 10, then 15 repetitions, twice daily. (Figure 8.14)

Straight Leg Raise

While lying on the floor on in bed, bend your knee slightly, or bend one knee to the chest if you have chronic back pain. Raise the other leg slowly while keeping the back firmly on the floor or bed. Raise your leg as high as you can, but stop if your back begins to arch. Hold and count to 6. Lower

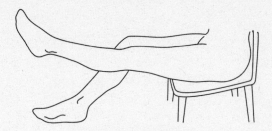

Figure 8.14

Knee and leg extension

your leg, and then repeat the stops for the opposite leg. Repeat for both legs, gradually increasing to 5, then 10, then 20 repetitions, twice daily. If you have severe pain with this or any exercise, stop immediately and talk to your doctor. (Figure 8.15)

Flexion

You can do this on the floor or in bed. Lie on your stomach and bend your knees as far as you can toward your back. Straighten your knee, then repeat, gradually increasing to 5, then 10, then 20 repetitions, twice daily.

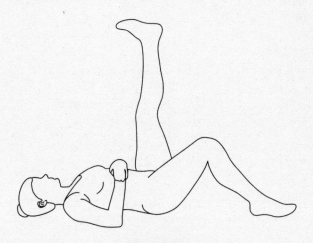

Figure 8.15

Straight leg raise

References and Supporting Research

Alexandersen, P., A. Toussaint, C. Christiansen, et al. "Ipriflavone in the treatment of postmenopausal osteoporosis: a randomized controlled trial." *Journal of the American Medical Association (JAMA)* 285 (2001): 1482.

American College of Rheumatology Ad Hoc Committee on Glucocorticoid-induced Osteoporosis. "Recommendations for the prevention and treatment of glucocorticoid-induced osteoporosis: 2001 update." *Arthritis and Rheumatism* 44 (2001): 1496–1503.

Burrows, M., A. M. Nevill, S. Bird, and D. Simpson. "Physiological factors associated with low bone mineral density in female endurance runners." *British Journal of Sports Medicine* 37 (February 2003): 67–71.

Cauley, J. A., J. Robbins, Z. Chen, et al. "Effects of estrogen plus progestin on risk of fracture and bone mineral density: the Women's Health Initiative randomized trial." *JAMA* 290 (2003): 1729–38.

Cumming, D. C. "Exercise-associated amenorrhea, low bone density, and estrogen replacement therapy." *Archives of Internal Medicine* 156 (1996): 2193.

Cummings, S. R., D. B. Karpf, F. Harris, et al. "Improvement in spine bone density and reduction in risk of vertebral fractures during treatment with antiresorptive drugs." *American Journal of Medicine* 112 (2002): 281.

Dawson-Hughes, B. "Bone loss accompanying medical therapies." *New England Journal of Medicine* 345 (September 2001): 989–91.

Ensrud K. E., T. L. Blackwell, C. M. Mangione, et al. "Central nervous system-active medications and risk for falls in older women." *Journal of the American Geriatric Society* 50 (October 2002): 1629–37.

Evans, J. G. "Drugs and falls in later life." *Lancet* 361 (2003): 448.

Feskanich D., W. Willett, and G. Colditz. "Walking and leisure-time activity and risk of hip fracture in postmenopausal women." *JAMA* 288 (2002): 2300–6.

Freedman, K. B., et al. "Treatment of osteoporosis: Are physicians missing an opportunity?" *Journal of Bone and Joint Surgery* 82-A (2000): 1063–70.

Friedlander, A. L., H. K. Genant, S. Sadowsky, et al. "A two-year program of aerobics and weight training enhances bone mineral density of young women." *Journal of Bone and Mineral Research* 10 (1995): 574.

Gerdhem, P., K. A. Ringsberg, K. Akesson, and K. J. Obrant. "Influence of muscle strength, physical activity and weight on bone mass in a population-based sample of 1,004 elderly women." *Osteoporosis International* 14 (2003): 768–72.

Gregg, E. W., J. A. Cauley, D. G. Seeley, et al. "Physical activity and osteoporotic fracture risk in older women." *Annals of Internal Medicine* 129 (1998): 81.

Hochberg, M. C., P. D. Ross, D. Black, et al. "Larger increases in bone mineral density during alendronate therapy are associated with a lower risk of new vertebral fractures in women with postmenopausal osteoporosis. Fracture Intervention Trial Research Group." *Arthritis and Rheumatology* 42 (1999): 1246.

Hosking, D., C. E. Chilvers, C. Christiansen, et al. "Prevention of bone loss with alendronate in postmenopausal women under 60 years of age." *New England Journal of Medicine* 338 (1998): 485.

Johnell, O., J. A. Kanis, A. Oden, et al. "Fracture risk following an osteoporotic fracture." *Osteoporosis International* (December 23, 2003). Available at: http://link.springer.de/link/service/journals/00198/.

Khosla, S., L. J. Melton, M. B. Dekutoski, et al. "Incidence of childhood distal forearm fractures over 30 years: a population-based study." *JAMA* 290 (2003): 1479–85.

Nelson, M. E., M. A. Fiatarone, C. M. Morganti, et al. "Effects of high-intensity strength training on multiple risk factors of osteoporotic fractures." *JAMA* 272 (1994): 1909.

Nyman, C., U. Pettersson, R. Lorentzon, et al. "Seasonal variation in bone mineral density of the calcaneous in a cohort of 2805 young men." Abstract P223SU. Presented at the World Congress of Osteoporosis, Lisbon, Portugal, May 2002.

NIH Consensus Conference. "NIH Consensus Development Panel on Osteoporosis. Prevention, Diagnosis, and Therapy." *JAMA* 285 (2001): 785.

Panneman, M. J., P. Lips, S. S. Sen, and R. M. Herings. "Undertreatment with anti-osteoporotic drugs after hospitalization for fracture." *Osteoporosis International* (November 13, 2003). Available at: http://dx.doi.org/10.1007/s00198-003-1544-7.

Rossouw, J. E., G. L. Anderson, and R. L. Prentice. "Risks and benefits of estrogen plus progestin in healthy postmenopausal women: principal results from the Women's Health Initiative randomized controlled trial." *JAMA* 288 (2002): 321.

Shumaker, S. A., C. Legault, S. R. Rapp, et al. for the WHIMS Investigators. "Estrogen plus progestin and the incidence of dementia and mild cognitive impairment in postmenopausal women. The Women's Health Initiative Memory Study: a randomized controlled trial." *JAMA* 289 (2003): 2651–62.

Sinaki, M., E. Itoi, H. W. Wahner, et al. "Stronger back muscles reduce the incidence of vertebral fractures: a prospective 10 year follow-up of postmenopausal women." *Bone* 30 (2002): 836–41.

Tucker, K. L., L. Troy, K. Morita, et al. "Presentation: carbonated beverage consumption and bone mineral density." Paper presented at the American Society for Bone and Mineral Research, Minneapolis, Minnesota, 25th annual meeting, September 19–23, 2003.

Turner, C. H. "Exercise as a therapy for osteoporosis: the drunk and the street lamp, revisited." *Bone* 23 (1998): 83.

U.S. Preventive Services Task Force. "Postmenopausal hormone replacement therapy for primary prevention of chronic conditions: recommendations and rationale." *Annals of Internal Medicine* 137 (2002): 834–39.

Support Websites

The American College of
Rheumatology
1800 Century Place, Suite 250
Atlanta, GA 30345
404-633-3777
http://www.rheumatology.org

The Arthritis Foundation
1314 Spring Street
Atlanta, GA 30309
800-283-7800
http://www.arthritis.org/

The Florida Osteoporosis Board
http://osteoporosisflorida.org

National Institute of Arthritis and
Musculoskeletal and Skin Diseases
One AMS Circle
Bethesda, MD 20892-3675
301-495-4484
http://www.nih.gov/niams/

National Institutes of Health—
Osteoporosis and Related Bone
Diseases
http://www.osteo.org

National Osteoporosis Foundation
1150 17th St. NW, #500
Washington, DC 20036-4603
800-223-9994
http://www.nof.org/

Tampa Medical Group, P.A.
http://www.tampamedicalgroup.com

SafeHip—Hip Protection Pads
http://www.hindso.suite.dk/

Acknowledgments

As with our previous health books, we have received generous assistance from a very select group of professionals.

For technical assistance, copyediting, and journal research, we thank the following: Robert G. Bruce Jr., P.M.P.; Linda McIlwain; Brittnye Bruce, M.S.; Claire Van Leuven Bruce, M.P.A.; Robert G. Bruce III; Hugh H. Cruse, M.P.H., M.S./M.I.S.; Michael McIlwain, D.M.D.; Christina Yarnoz McIlwain; Ashley Bruce Trehan, and Sunjay Daniel Trehan.

For excellent medical line art and design, we thank James Russell, M.S.

We thank our agent, Denise Marcil, whose personal enthusiasm for a groundbreaking book on reversing osteopenia fueled our writing of this guide.

Last, we acknowledge our editors at Holt, Deborah Brody and Lisa Considine, who believe in the power of the written word for health education.

Index

Note: Page numbers in italics indicate box text.

About the Authors

HARRIS H. MCILWAIN, M.D., a board-certified rheumatologist, is the founder of the Tampa Medical Group. He has served as chairman of the Florida Osteoporosis Board since its inception five years ago. *Town and Country* has twice named him one of its Best Doctors in America.

LAURA MCILWAIN CRUSE, M.D., and KIMBERLY LYNN MCILWAIN, M.D., are rheumatologists and board-certified internists in Florida.

DEBRA FULGHUM BRUCE, Ph.D., has written more than 2,500 articles and 65 books on various health topics.